Basic Medical Terminology

Fourth Edition

J. Patrick Fisher
Retired Instructor
Medical Secretary Program
Elkhart Area Career Center
Elkhart, Indiana

◆

Editorial Consultant

Nancy P. Hutzell
Kaw Area Technical School
Topeka, Kansas

GLENCOE

Macmillan/McGraw-Hill

New York, New York   Columbus, Ohio   Mission Hills, California   Peoria, Illinois

Library of Congress Cataloging-in-Publication Data

Fisher, J. Patrick.
Basic medical terminology / J. Patrick Fisher; editorial consultant, Nancy P. Hutzell.—4th ed.
p. cm.
Includes index.
ISBN 0-02-800875-8 (text with study tapes: pbk.).—ISBN 0-02-800876-6 (instructor's guide).—ISBN 0-02-800877-4 (lab tapes)
1. Medicine—Terminology. I. Hutzell, Nancy P. II. Title.
[DNLM: 1. Nomenclature. W 15 F534b]
R123.F5 1993
610'.14—dc20
DNLM/DLC 92-48811
for Library of Congress CIP

Send all inquiries to:
GLENCOE DIVISION
Macmillan/McGraw-Hill
936 Eastwind Drive
Westerville, OH 43081

ISBN 0-02-800875-8 (Text with Study Tapes)
ISBN 0-02-800876-6 (Instructor's Guide)
ISBN 0-02-800877-4 (Lab Tapes)

Printed in the United States of America

2 3 4 5 6 7 8 9 POH 99 98 97 96 95 94 93

PREFACE

Health care is a team effort that involves the talents and abilities of people in a variety of health occupations, including medical assistants, respiratory therapists, x-ray technicians, medical record technicians, and medical secretaries. Each member of the health team must be a skilled technician. Each must be able to carry out the increasingly complex techniques required by modern patient care and must have a good, basic knowledge of the medical field as a whole.

This textbook is designed to develop one of the most basic skills needed in the allied health fields, a knowledge of medical terminology. It contains the clear, concise information that you need to build a foundation for competence in your chosen field.

Since its first publication in 1976, *Basic Medical Terminology* has enjoyed wide use in a variety of allied health programs. The Fourth Edition retains the clear, simple format that appealed to users of earlier editions. The terms are organized according to body systems so the learning program can be more easily correlated with a basic anatomy course. All terms are pronounced on the accompanying audio cassettes and reviewed in extensive practice lessons to build solid skills in spelling and pronunciation. The tape and workbook format is particularly well-suited to self-paced individual learning programs, but it is also readily adaptable to standard lecture and discussion classes.

INTRODUCTION

Anyone entering a health occupation must have a working knowledge of basic medical terminology. Medical terms may seem very complicated at first glance, but they are not difficult to master if broken down into meaningful parts.

In this course, you will be given the various parts (word elements) that make up medical terms and will learn how those word parts are put together to form medical terms.

For example, in Lesson 1 you will learn the combining form, *cardi(o)*, a word part that refers to the heart. It is called a *combining form* because it consists of a word root, *cardi,* plus an extra vowel, *o,* that allows the root to be combined with other word parts. The extra vowel, or *combining vowel,* makes combinations of word parts easier to pronounce. It is usually an *o*, but sometimes may be an *a* or an *i*. In this text, we show the combining vowel in parentheses, as in *cardi(o)*, *neur(o)*, etc.

Words roots usually refer to parts of the body. *Prefixes* and *suffixes* are added to these word roots to extend or change their meaning. Prefixes are attached *before* the root. They usually denote amounts, positions, and various kinds of relationships. Suffixes are attached *behind* the root and denote action about the root (e.g., pain, inflammation). Roots may be combined with several prefixes or suffixes or with other roots.

Let's look at some examples. The combining form *cost(o)* refers to the ribs. If we add the prefix *inter-*("between") to the beginning of the word root and the suffix *-al*("pertaining to") to the end, we have the medical term *intercostal*. It means "pertaining to the area between the ribs." The combining form *neur(o)* (referring to the nerves) may take the suffix *-itis* ("inflammation") to become the term *neuritis*, meaning "inflammation of the nerves." The word *cardiovascular* shows how two combining forms, *cardi(o)* and *vascul(o)*, may be put together. Since the root *vascul(o)* refers to vessels and the suffix *-ar* means "pertaining to," *cardiovascular* means "pertaining to the heart and blood vessels."

Notice that prefixes are written with hyphens following them *(hyper-, pre-, quadri-)*. Suffixes are shown with a hyphen preceding them *(-oma, -algia, -osis)*. We show them this way throughout the text, but we will refer to them simply as "word parts" or "word elements" from this point on. The important thing is to remember their meanings, not whether they happen to be prefixes or suffixes or word roots.

Once you have learned the basic word elements, most of the medical terms you come across can be broken down and understood immediately. In a few cases, you may need the help of a medical dictionary to understand the full meaning of the term. For example, you might know that *ankyl(o)* means "crooked" and *gloss(o)* means "the tongue," but you may have to check *ankyloglossia* in a medical dictionary to understand that it means "tongue-tied."

Dictionary Basis

A medical dictionary also will be useful for checking the pronunciation of words. *Dorland's Illustrated Medical Dictionary* was used as the primary pronunciation authority for this course, but whatever medical dictionary your instructor makes available will serve the purpose. You will discover, as you go through the course, that some terms have more than one correct pronunciation. In such cases, pronunciation is mainly a matter of personal choice or local custom.

In the workbook, you will find phonetic respellings for new terms. These show only how the consonants are pronounced and which syllables are accented. For more detailed information on the pronunciation of vowels and on pronunciation variations, consult the dictionary. You should become familiar with the pronunciation key in your dictionary. This key is located in the front of the dictionary or at the bottom of each page. It will show you how to interpret the pronunciation respelling for the word you are looking up.

Course Organization

This course contains 71 lessons, organized into 14 sections, with corresponding Lab Tapes and Study Tapes for each lesson. The first 10 sections are devoted to the body systems (cardiovascular, respiratory and so on). Section 11 discusses numbers, amounts and colors; Section 12 is devoted to the medical specialties; Section 13 covers basic dental terms that will introduce you to this subject area; and Section 14 presents common drugs and their definitions.

The first four or five lessons in each section are Terminology Presentation. For each of these, the Lab Tap and the workbook pages will present a number of combining forms and word parts, so that you can see how these word elements appear in different medical terms. The Study Tapes at the back of this text will provide another means of reinforcement.

The last lesson in each section is a Terminology Review. These reviews present words that are made up of word elements you have learned in the previous lessons. You will divide these words into their familiar parts and find out what they mean. You will then test yourself on how well you remember the word parts from that section. When you feel that you know the word parts thoroughly, you can take the test.

Glossary and Index

In the back of the workbook you will find a glossary and a comprehensive index. The Glossary gives you an alphabetical listing of each word part and term together with its definition. You can use the Index to find the page number of word elements and terms. Your instructor may make available a copy of the Instructor's Guide. This guide contains answer keys you can use to correct your own tests. You can find out immediately which words and word elements you must study further before proceeding to the next section. If you have any difficulties, consult with your instructor or check your dictionary.

There are three areas you must concentrate on when you learn a new word element or medical term; pronunciation (provided on the recordings), spelling, and meaning (as found in the workbook). Correct pronunciation, correct spelling, and precise meaning are all essential to your use and understanding of medical terminology on the job.

This course is designed so you can work at the pace that is best for you. You can repeat a lesson as often as you wish to become thoroughly familiar with the word parts and terms. You can refer back to earlier lessons whenever you feel it is necessary. If you carefully follow the instructions in both the audio and the workbook sections, and if you take the time to learn each group of new terms thoroughly, you will have a solid working knowledge of basic medical terminology by the end of the course.

Now you are ready to begin. Listen carefully to the introduction presented on the first Lab Tape. Read the instructions for Lesson 1 and follow each direction as given.

Contents

SECTION 1

Cardiovascular System

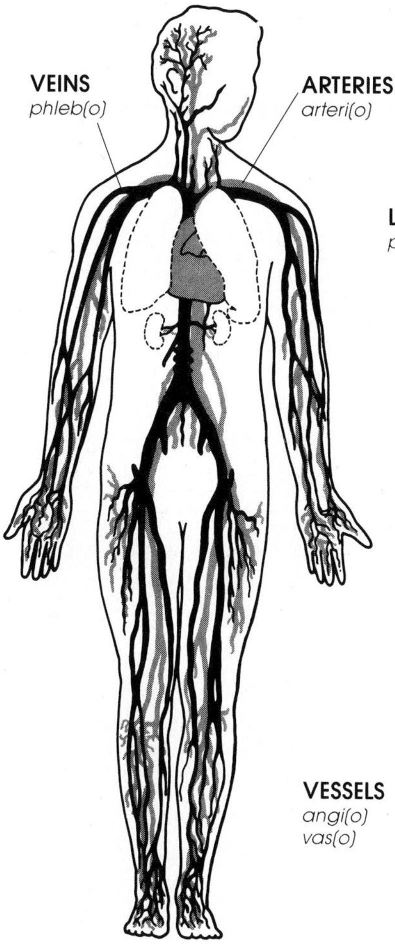

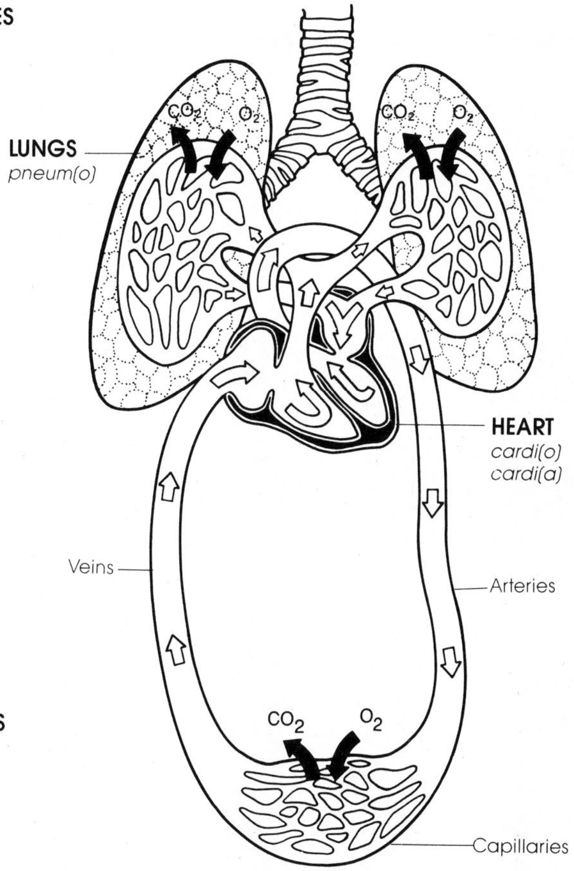

BLOOD CLOT
thromb(o)

PULSE or BLOOD PRESSURE
sphygm(o)

CARDIOVASCULAR SYSTEM

Orientation

The cardiovascular system consists of the heart and blood vessels. The heart is a hollow muscle about the size of a fist. It acts as a pump that forces blood to circulate, under pressure, through a series of tubes, the blood vessels. The heart is one of the strongest organs in the human body. It does an incredible amount of work in the human life span. With an average rate of 70 to 80 beats per minute, it will beat more than 2½ billion times in 70 years. An average adult heart pumps about 4,000 gallons of blood a day.

The heart is located between the lungs, somewhat to the left of the center of the body. There are three layers in the heart wall. The first is the endocardium, the membrane which lines the inside of the heart. The valves of the heart are also composed of this material. The second and thickest layer is the myocardium; the heart muscle. The outermost layer is the epicardium. Enclosing the heart is the pericardial sac, which is lined with pericardium.

Blood is pumped throughout the body to deliver food and oxygen to the body cells. It is pumped through the lungs where carbon dioxide is removed and oxygen is picked up before recirculating. The blood then moves through the body where it provides oxygen to the cells and picks up waste material such as carbon dioxide. Blood pressure is determined by the force of the heartbeat and the condition of the walls of the vessels. The heart is the pump. The active phase of contraction or pumping is known as systole and is followed by the resting phase known as diastole, thus the terms *systolic pressure* and *diastolic pressure*. The heart rate and the muscles in the vessel walls are controlled by the nervous system.

There are two types of vessels, arteries and veins. The arteries carry blood away from the heart and the veins return the blood to the heart. Arteries and veins are connected by thin-walled vessels called capillaries. These capillaries allow transfer of substances between the blood and body cells.

Abnormal heart sounds are called murmurs and are due to faulty action of the valves of the heart. If the valves fail to close tightly and blood leaks back, a murmur is heard. Another condition causing an abnormal sound is the narrowing, or stenosis, of the valve orifice, or opening.

LESSON 1

Terminology Presentation

Listen to the Lab Tape provided by your instructor, and you will hear the words presented in this lesson. Read the words as they are said, noticing spelling and pronunciation. The recording will tell you when the presentation for this lesson is completed and will give you any further instructions. Do not go on to the next recorded lesson until you have completed Lesson 1 and feel that you know the words and word parts that have been presented.

• • • ▶ ***Start Audio***

cardi(o) or ***cardi(a)*** a combining form denoting the heart

WORD	WORD PART	DEFINITION	ANSWER
1. carditis (kar-di'tis)	-itis	inflammation	1. ____________
2. cardiology (kar-de-ol'o-je)	-(o)logy	study of, science of	2. ____________
3. cardiac (kar'de-ak)	-ac	resembling, pertaining to	3. ____________
4. cardiograph (kar'de-o-graf')	-graph	an instrument for recording	4. ____________
5. cardiogram (kar'de-o-gram')	-gram	something recorded	5. ____________
6. cardiomegaly (kar'de-o-meg'ah-le)	-megaly	enlargement	6. ____________
7. cardiospasm (kar'de-o-spazm')	-spasm	contraction	7. ____________
8. cardiologist (kar-de-ol'o-jist)	-(o)logist	specialist	8. ____________
9. bradycardia (brad'e-kar'de-ah)	brady	slow	9. ____________
10. cardiopathy (kar'de-op'ah-the)	-pathy	disease	10. ____________

11. pericarditis (per'i-kar-di'tis)	peri -itis	around inflamation	**11.** ____________
12. tachycardia (tak'e-kar'de-ah)	tachy	fast	**12.** ____________
13. cardiorrhaphy (kar'de-or'ah-fe)	-rrhaphy	suture, surgical repair	**13.** ____________
14. endocarditis (en'do-kar-di'tis)	endo -itis	within inflammation	**14.** ____________
15. cardiotomy (kar'de-ot'o-me)	-tomy	incision, cutting into	**15.** ____________

■ • • • *Stop Audio at Tone*

Study the 15 words and word parts for this lesson. Practice each word several times, checking your spelling and repeating the meaning to yourself. Listen to the recording and pronounce the words as many times as necessary. When you feel that you know the words and word parts well, you are ready to go on to the next step.

Use a sheet of paper to cover all columns except the Answer Column on the previous page. The words you have learned will be presented again on the recording. As each word is pronounced, write it in the space provided in the Answer Column.

• • • ▶ *Start Audio*

After stopping the tape player, check the words you have written against the words in the left-hand column. If any words are misspelled, practice writing them correctly. When you feel that you know and understand the words and word parts, go on to the Terminology Practice.

PRACTICE

Name ______________________ Date ______________ Errors ________

LESSON 1: TERMINOLOGY PRACTICE

Without looking at your previous work, write the word that is described by each definition.

cardi(o) or *cardi(a)*

DEFINITION	TERM
1. Excessive rapidity in the action of the heart, usually in the pulse rate	______________
2. Inflammation within the heart	______________
3. Surgical incision into the heart	______________
4. A specialist in treating heart disorders	______________
5. A contraction of the heart	______________
6. A disease of the heart	______________
7. An instrument for recording the heart rate	______________
8. Pertaining to the heart	______________
9. Suture or surgical repair of the heart	______________
10. The recording of the heart's movements	______________
11. The science or study of the heart	______________
12. Inflammation of the membrane around the heart	______________
13. Abnormally slow heartbeat	______________
14. Inflammation of the heart	______________
15. Enlargement of the heart	______________

Check your answers against the word and definition lists on the first page of this lesson. If you have any errors, count them and write the number in the blank at the top of the page. Practice any missed or misspelled words in the space provided. Sign your work and give it to your instructor. You are now ready for the next lesson.

PRACTICE

LESSON 2

Terminology Presentation

Listen to the Lab Tape provided by your instructor, and you will hear the words presented in this lesson. Read the words as they are said, noticing spelling and pronunciation. The recording will tell you when the presentation for this lesson is completed and will give you any further instructions. Do not go on to the next recorded lesson until you have completed Lesson 2 and feel that you know the words and word parts that have been presented.

• • • ▶ *Start Audio*

phleb(o) a word element denoting a vein or the veins

WORD	WORD PART	DEFINITION	ANSWER
1. phlebotomy (fle-bot′o-me)	-tomy	incision, cutting into	1. ______
2. phlebitis (fle-bi′tis)	-itis	inflammation	2. ______
3. phlebodynamics (fleb′o-di-nam′iks)	-dynamics	force	3. ______
4. phleborrhagia (fleb′o-ra′je-ah)	-rrhagia	excessive flow, bleeding	4. ______
5. phlebosclerosis (fleb′o-skle-ro′sis)	-sclerosis	hardening	5. ______
6. phlebostenosis (fleb′o-ste-no′sis)	-stenosis	narrowing	6. ______
7. phleboplasty (fleb′o-plas′te)	-plasty	plastic surgery	7. ______
8. phleborrhaphy (fle-bor′ah-fe)	-rrhaphy	suture, surgical repair	8. ______

art or ***arteri(o)*** a word element denoting the arteries

WORD	WORD PART	DEFINITION	ANSWER
9. arteriorrhexis (ar-te′re-o-rek′sis)	-rrhexis	rupture	9. ______

10. arteriosclerosis (ar-te're-o-skle-ro'sis)	-sclerosis	hardening	10. ________
11. arteritis (ar'te-ri'tis)	-itis	inflammation	11. ________
12. arterial (ar-te're-al)	-al	of, pertaining to	12. ________
13. arteriopathy (ar'te-re-op'ah-the)	-pathy	disease	13. ________
14. arteriectasis (ar'te-re-ek'tah-sis)	-ectasis	dilatation, expansion	14. ________
15. arteriostrepsis (ar-te're-o-strep'sis)	-strepsis	a twisting	15. ________
16. arteriorrhaphy (ar-te're-or'ah-fe)	-rrhaphy	suture, surgical repair	16. ________

■ • • • *Stop Audio at Tone*

Study the 16 words and word parts for this lesson. Practice each word several times, checking your spelling and repeating the meaning to yourself. Listen to the recording and pronounce the words as many times as necessary. When you feel that you know the words and word parts well, you are ready to go on to the next step.

Use a sheet of paper to cover all columns except the Answer Column on the previous page. The words you have learned will be presented again on the recording. As each word is pronounced, write it in the space provided in the Answer Column.

• • • ▶ *Start Audio*

After stopping the tape player, check the words you have written against the words in the left-hand column. If any words are misspelled, practice writing them correctly. When you feel that you know and understand the words and word parts, go on to the Terminology Practice.

PRACTICE

____

____

____

____

____

____

Name ______________________ Date ______________ Errors ________

LESSON 2: TERMINOLOGY PRACTICE

Without looking at your previous work, write the word that is described by each definition.

phleb(o) or *arteri(a)*

DEFINITION	TERM
1. Hardening of the arteries	______________
2. Suture or repair of a vein	______________
3. A disease of an artery	______________
4. Dilatation of an artery	______________
5. Excessive bleeding from a vein	______________
6. Twisting of an artery to stop bleeding	______________
7. Hardening of the walls of the veins	______________
8. Suture or repair of an artery	______________
9. Laws and principles governing blood pressure	______________
10. Incision into a vein	______________
11. Inflammation of a vein	______________
12. Rupture of an artery	______________
13. Narrowing or constricting of a vein	______________
14. Inflammation of an artery	______________
15. Plastic surgery for repair of a vein	______________
16. Of or pertaining to an artery	______________

Check your answers against the word and definition lists on the first page of this lesson. If you have any errors, count them and write the number in the blank at the top of the page. Practice any missed or misspelled words in the space provided. Sign your work and give it to your instructor. You are now ready for the next lesson.

PRACTICE

LESSON 3

Terminology Presentation

Listen to the Lab Tape provided by your instructor, and you will hear the words presented in this lesson. Read the words as they are said, noticing spelling and pronunciation. The recording will tell you when the presentation for this lesson is completed and will give you any further instructions. Do not go on to the next recorded lesson until you have completed Lesson 3 and feel that you know the words and word parts that have been presented.

• • • ▶ *Start Audio*

thromb(o) a combining form indicating a blood clot, or thrombus

WORD	WORD PART	DEFINITION	ANSWER
1. thrombocyte (throm′bo-site)	-cyte	cell	1. ________
2. thrombopoiesis (throm′bo-poi-e′sis)	-poiesis	form, formation	2. ________
3. thrombosis (throm-bo′sis)	-osis	condition, process, increase, disease	3. ________
4. thrombogenic (throm′bo-jen′ik)	-gen, genesis -ic	producing pertaining to	4. ________
5. thromboarteritis (throm′bo-ar′ter-i′tis)	-arteri(o) -itis	arteries inflammation	5. ________
6. thromboclasis (throm-bok′lah-sis)	-clasis	break, fracture	6. ________
7. thrombectomy (throm-bek′to-me)	-ectomy	excision, removal	7. ________
8. thromboid (throm′boid)	-oid	like, resembling	8. ________
9. thrombocytosis (throm′bo-si-to′sis)	cyt(o) -osis	cell condition, process, increase, disease	9. ________
10. thrombocytopenia (throm′bo-si′to-pe′ne-ah)	-cyt(o) -penia	cell decrease	10. ________

11. thrombophlebitis (throm′bo-fle-bi′tis)	phleb(o) -itis	vein inflammation	**11.** ________
12. thrombopathy (throm-bop′ah-the)	-pathy	disease	**12.** ________

■ • • • *Stop Audio at Tone*

Study the 12 words and word parts for this lesson. Practice each word several times, checking your spelling and repeating the meaning to yourself. Listen to the recording and pronounce the words as many times as necessary. When you feel that you know the words and word parts well, you are ready to go on to the next step.

Use a sheet of paper to cover all columns except the Answer Column on the previous page. The words you have learned will be presented again on the recording. As each word is pronounced, write it in the space provided in the Answer Column.

• • • ▶ *Start Audio*

After stopping the tape player, check the words you have written against the words in the left-hand column. If any words are mispelled, practice writing them correctly. When you feel that you know and understand the words and word parts, go on to the Terminology Practice.

PRACTICE

Name ______________________ Date ______________ Errors ________

LESSON 3: TERMINOLOGY PRACTICE

Without looking at your previous work, write the word that is described by each definition.

thromb(o)

DEFINITION	TERM
1. Inflammation of an artery with a clot present	______________
2. An unusually large number of thrombocytes (platelets) in the blood	______________
3. A clotting cell	______________
4. Disease involving the clotting cells	______________
5. The formation of clots or thrombi	______________
6. Decrease in the number of clotting cells	______________
7. A condition in which a thrombus is present	______________
8. Inflammation of a vein in which a clot or thrombus is present	______________
9. The breaking up or dissolution of a thrombus	______________
10. Producing a clot or thrombus	______________
11. Like or resembling a clot	______________
12. Removal or excision of a thrombus	______________

Check your answers against the word and definition lists on the first page of this lesson. If you have any errors, count them and write the number in the blank at the top of the page. Practice any missed or misspelled words on the next page. Sign your work and give it to your instructor. You are now ready for the next lesson.

PRACTICE

LESSON

4 Terminology Presentation

Listen to the Lab Tape provided by by your instructor, and you will hear the words presented in this lesson. Read the words as they are said, noticing spelling and pronunciation. The recording will tell you when the presentation for this lesson is completed and will give you any further instructions. Do not go on to the next recorded lesson until you have completed Lesson 4 and feel that you know the words and word parts that have been presented.

sphygm(o) a word part denoting the pulse or blood pressure

WORD	WORD PART	DEFINITION	ANSWER
1. sphygmogram (sfig′mo-gram)	-gram	something recorded	1. ______
2. sphygmoid (sfig′moid)	-oid	like, resembling	2. ______
3. sphygmology (sfig-mol′o-je)	-(o)logy	study of, science of	3. ______
4. sphygmopalpation (sfig′mo-pal-pa′shun)	-palpation	feeling	4. ______
5. sphygmomanometer (sfig′mo-mah-nom′e-ter)	mano -meter	thin, scanty measure	5. ______
6. sphygmoscopy (sfig-mos′ko-pe)	-scopy	examine	6. ______

vas(o) a word part denoting a vessel or duct

WORD	WORD PART	DEFINITION	ANSWER
7. vasomotor (vas-o-mo′tor)	-motor	producing movement	7. ______
8. vasosection (vas′o-sek′shun)	sect	cut	8. ______
9. vasectomy (vah-sek′to-me)	-ectomy	excision, removal	9. ______

10. vasorrhaphy (vas-or'ah-fe)	-rrhaphy	suture, surgical repair	10. ________
11. vasography (vah-sog'rah-fe)	-graphy	recording	11. ________
12. vasospasm (vas'o-spazm)	-spasm	contraction	12. ________

■ • • • *Stop Audio at Tone*

Study the 12 words and word parts for this lesson. Practice each word several times, checking your spelling and repeating the meaning to yourself. Listen to the recording and pronounce the words as many times as necessary. When you feel that you know the words and word parts well, you are ready to go on to the next step.

Use a sheet of paper to cover all columns except the Answer Column on the previous page. The words you have learned will be presented again on the recording. As each word is pronounced, write it in the space provided in the Answer Column.

• • • ▶ *Start Audio*

After stopping the tape player, check the words you have written against the words in the left-hand column. If any words are misspelled, practice writing them correctly. When you feel that you know and understand the words and word parts, go on to the Terminology Practice.

PRACTICE

Name ______________________ Date ______________ Errors ________

LESSON 4: TERMINOLOGY PRACTICE

Without looking at your previous work, write the word that is described by each definition.

sphygm(o) and *vas(o)*

DEFINITION	TERM
1. The study or science of what is known on the pulse	______________
2. Suture of a vessel or the ductus deferens	______________
3. Examination of the pulse	______________
4. Surgical removal of the ductus deferens, or a portion of it	______________
5. Contraction of a vessel	______________
6. The cutting of a vessel	______________
7. Palpating or feeling the pulse	______________
8. An instrument for measuring the blood pressure	______________
9. Record or tracing of the pulse	______________
10. Affecting the movement and size of a vessel	______________
11. X-ray picture, or roentgenography, of the blood vessels	______________
12. Like or resembling the pulse	______________

Check your answers against the word and definition lists on the first page of this lesson. If you have any errors, count them and write the number in the blank at the top of the page. Practice any missed or misspelled words on the next page. Sign your work and give it to your instructor. You may now go on to the next lesson.

PRACTICE

Name ______________________ Date ______________ Errors ________

LESSON 5 | TERMINOLOGY REVIEW FOR TEST 1

This is a review of the word parts you have learned in the preceding four lessons. Some of the medical terms listed below may be new, but they are made up of word parts that you have already learned. Read the words below as they are pronounced on the Lab Tape. As you listen, notice the familiar word parts which make them up.

• • • ▸ *Start Audio*

WORD	WORD PART	MEANING OF WORD PART
1. arteriosclerosis	arteri(o)	______________
(ar-te′re-o′skle-ro′sis)	-sclerosis	______________
arteriosclerosis	______________	
2. phleborrhaphy	phleb(o)	______________
(fle-bor′ah-fe)	-rraphy	______________
phleborrhaphy	______________	
3. thrombocytopenia	thromb(o)	______________
(throm′bo-si′to-pe′ne-ah)	cyt(o)	______________
	-penia	______________
thrombocytopenia	______________	
4. phlebectomy	phleb(o)	______________
(fle-bek′to-me)	-ectomy	______________
phlebectomy	______________	
5. sphygmogram	sphygm(o)	______________
(sfig′mo-gram)	-gram	______________
sphygmogram	______________	
6. arteriospasm	arteri(o)	______________
(ar-te′re-o-spazm′)	-spasm	______________
arteriospasm	______________	
7. cardiorrhaphy	cardi(o)	______________
(kar′de-or′ah-fe)	-rrhaphy	______________
cardiorrhaphy	______________	
8. thromboid	thromb(o)	______________
(throm′boid)	-oid	______________
thromboid	______________	

9. sphygmopalpation (sfig'mo-pal-pa'shun)
sphygm(o) ______________________
-palpation ______________________
sphygmopalpation ______________________________________

10. vasosection (vas'o-sek'shun)
vas(o) ______________________
sect ______________________
vasosection ______________________________________

11. tachycardia (tak'e-kar-de-ah)
tachy ______________________
-cardia ______________________
tachycardia ______________________________________

12. arteriectasis (ar'te-re-ek'tah-sis)
arteri(o) ______________________
-ectasis ______________________
arteriectasis ______________________________________

13. thrombopoiesis (throm'bo-poi-e'sis)
thromb(o) ______________________
-poiesis ______________________
thrombopoiesis ______________________________________

14. sphygmomanometer (sfig'mo-mah-nom'e-ter)
sphygm(o) ______________________
-mano ______________________
-meter ______________________
sphygmomanometer ______________________________________

15. vasectomy (vah-sek'to-me)
vas(o) ______________________
-ectomy ______________________
vasectomy ______________________________________

■ • • • *Stop Audio at Tone*

On the lines provided, fill in the meanings of as many of the word parts as you can from memory. Then, use the previous lessons or a medical dictionary to look up any definitions you could not remember. Fill them in. On a separate piece of paper, practice writing the word parts and their meanings. Pay special attention to any which you had trouble remembering. Be sure to check your spelling.

When you have defined and reviewed all the word parts, write a definition for each whole word on the line provided. Check your definitions in the Glossary or a medical dictionary and make any needed corrections. Practice the words on a separate sheet of paper until you are sure that you know them. Then go on to the Extra Credit Review (if your instructor assigns it) or Test 1.

Name ______________________ Date ______________ Errors ________

LESSON 5 — EXTRA CREDIT REVIEW

This Extra Credit Review should be done at the discretion of your instructor. If you are instructed to complete this portion of the Review, turn it in to your instructor when you are finished.

PART A

Each phrase below defines one of the words you have just studied. Without looking at your previous work, fill in the word that matches each definition.

DEFINITION	TERM
1. Dilatation of an artery	______________
2. Suture of a vein	______________
3. Contraction of an artery	______________
4. The formation of clots or thrombi	______________
5. Decrease in the number of clotting cells	______________
6. Record or tracing of the pulse	______________
7. Excessive rapidity in the action of the heart—especially the pulse rate	______________
8. Palpating or feeling the pulse	______________
9. The cutting of a vessel	______________
10. Excision or removal of a vein	______________
11. Surgical removal of the ductus deferens, or a portion of it	______________
12. Like or resembling a clot	______________
13. An instrument for measuring the blood pressure	______________
14. Suture or surgical repair of the heart	______________
15. Hardening of the artery or arteries	______________

PART B

Match the following terms with the definitions given. Place the correct letter of the term to the left of the definition.

DEFINITION	TERM
______ **16.** Abnormally slow heartbeat	a. thromboclasis
______ **17.** The laws and principles governing blood pressure	b. arteriorrhexis
______ **18.** The study or science of what is known of the pulse	c. phlebodynamics
______ **19.** Rupture of an artery	d. thrombocytopenia
______ **20.** Affecting the movement and size of a vessel	e. bradycardia
______ **21.** Hardening of a vein	f. sphygmology
______ **22.** Enlargement of the heart	g. vasomotor
______ **23.** Decrease in the number of clotting cells	h. phlebosclerosis
______ **24.** A twisting of an artery for the arrest of hemorrhage	i. cardiomegaly
______ **25.** The breaking up or dissolution of a thrombus	j. arteriostrepsis

You may now go on to Test 1.

SECTION

2 Musculoskeletal System

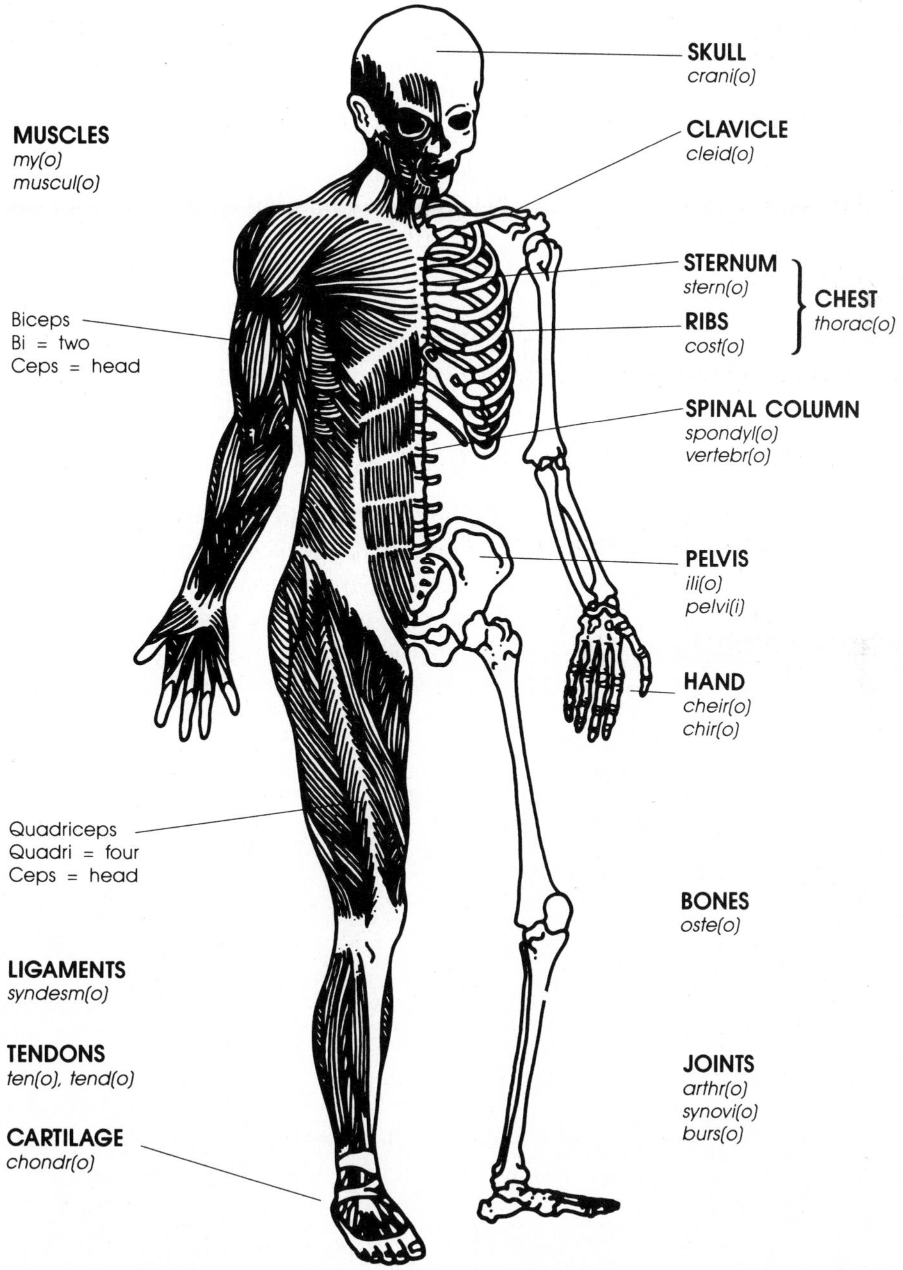

SKULL
crani(o)
MUSCLES
my(o)
muscul(o)
CLAVICLE
cleid(o)
STERNUM
stern(o)
CHEST
thorac(o)
Biceps
Bi = two
Ceps = head
RIBS
cost(o)
SPINAL COLUMN
spondyl(o)
vertebr(o)
PELVIS
ili(o)
pelvi(i)
HAND
cheir(o)
chir(o)
Quadriceps
Quadri = four
Ceps = head
BONES
oste(o)
LIGAMENTS
syndesm(o)
TENDONS
ten(o), tend(o)
JOINTS
arthr(o)
synovi(o)
burs(o)
CARTILAGE
chondr(o)

MUSCULOSKELETAL SYSTEM

Orientation

Bones, muscles, and joints make up the musculoskeletal system. This system gives the body a supporting framework, protection for vital organs, and the ability to move. Bones are made up of a special type of connective tissue, which is hard due to deposits of the mineral calcium. Bones are divided into four classes according to their shape: long, short, flat, and irregular. Almost all bones are covered on the outside by a membrane called periosteum, which contains many nerve fibers and lymphatics. Inside most bones is a spongy type of tissue, bone marrow, which manufactures several different types of blood cells.

At the places where bones are connected, called joints, the bone ends are lined with cartilage. As strong bands of connective tissue, the ligaments help to hold bones in place. Certain joints have a saclike structure called a bursa surrounding them that prevents friction between moving parts, such as tendons and bones. Common bursal locations are at the elbow, knee, and shoulder joint.

The three kinds of muscle tissue are skeletal, smooth, and cardiac. Skeletal muscles may be regarded as organs since they are made up of muscle and connective tissue. These muscles give shape and form to the body. Because they operate at one's will, they are known as voluntary muscles. Smooth and cardiac muscles are involuntary muscles. They generally work without direction from the individual. The muscles of the heart, digestive tract, and blood vessels are involuntary muscles.

Most muscles have two or more attachments to the bones. The method of attachment varies. In some parts of the body, the connective tissue within the muscle is attached to the periosteum of the bone. These attachments are called tendons. Connective tissues that are broad and sheetlike are known as aponeuroses, and they serve to attach muscle to bone or other tissue. Some muscles attach to cartilage. Cartilage is a dense connective tissue found in several regions of the adult body. Some of these regions are the nasal septum, larynx, trachea, bronchi, external ear, and covering the surfaces of movable joints.

LESSON 6

Terminology Presentation

Listen to the Lab Tape provided by your instructor, and you will hear the words presented in this lesson. Read the words as they are said, noticing spelling and pronunciation. The recording will tell you when the presentation for this lesson is completed and will give you any further instructions. Do not go on to the next recorded lesson until you have completed Lesson 6 and feel that you know the words and word parts that have been presented.

••• ▸ ***Start Audio***

cheir(o) or ***chir(o)*** a word element denoting the hands

WORD	WORD PART	DEFINITION	ANSWER
1. cheirarthritis (ki′rar-thri′tis)	arthr(o) -itis	joints inflammation	1. ________
2. cheiropodalgia (ki′ro-po-dal′je-ah)	pod -algia	foot pain	2. ________
3. cheirobrachialgia (ki′ro-bra′ke-al′je-ah)	brachi(o) -algia	arm pain	3. ________
4. chiropractic (ki′ro-prak′tik)	pract -ic	to do, to practice pertaining to	4. ________
5. cheiroplasty (ki′ro-plas′te)	-plasty	plastic surgery	5. ________
6. cheirospasm (ki′ro-spazm)	-spasm	contraction	6. ________
7. cheiromegaly (ki-ro-meg′ah-le)	-megaly	enlargement	7. ________

oste(o) a word element denoting the bones

WORD	WORD PART	DEFINITION	ANSWER
8. osteofibroma (os′te-o-fi-bro′mah)	fibr(o) -oma	fibrous tumor	8. ________
9. osteoporosis (os′te-o-po-ro′sis)	poros -osis	pore, opening condition	9. ________

10. osteogenesis (os′te-o-jen′e-sis)	-genesis	producing	10. ______
11. osteoclasis (os-te-ok′lah-sis)	-clasis	break, fracture	11. ______
12. osteohypertrophy (os′te-o-hi-per′tro-fe)	hyper -trophy	above, over abundant nourishment	12. ______
13. osteomalacia (os′te-o-mah-la′she-ah)	-malacia	softening	13. ______
14. osteolysis (os′te-ol′i-sis)	-(o)lysis	dissolve, break down	14. ______
15. osteitis (os′te-i′tis)	-itis	inflammation	15. ______

■ • • • *Stop Audio at Tone*

Study the 15 words and word parts for this lesson. Practice each word several times, checking your spelling and repeating the meaning to yourself. Listen to the recording and pronounce the words as many times as necessary. When you feel that you know the words and word parts well, you are ready to go to the next step.

Use a sheet of paper to cover all columns except the Answer Column on the previous page. The words you have learned will be repeated again on the recording. As each word is pronounced, write it in the space provided in the Answer Column.

• • • ▶ *Start Audio*

After stopping the tape player, check the words you have written against the words in the left-hand column. If any words are misspelled, practice writing them correctly. When you feel that you know and understand the words and word parts, go on to the Terminology Practice.

PRACTICE

Name ______________________ Date ______________ Errors ________

LESSON 6: TERMINOLOGY PRACTICE

Without looking at your previous work, write the word that is described by each definition.

cheir(o), chir(o), and *oste(o)*

DEFINITION	TERM
1. Enlargement of the hands	____________
2. A condition characterized by overgrowth of bones	____________
3. Surgical fracture or refracture of a bone	____________
4. Pain in the hands and feet	____________
5. Producing bone	____________
6. Inflammation of the joints of the hands	____________
7. Painful condition of the hand and arm	____________
8. Inflammation of a bone	____________
9. A system of therapeutics which attempts to restore normal function of the body by manipulation of the human body	____________
10. Contraction of the hand	____________
11. Tumor composed of osseous or fibrous material	____________
12. Reduction in the quantity of bone or atrophy of skeletal tissue	____________
13. Softening of the bone	____________
14. Softening, destruction, and absorption of bony tissue	____________
15. Plastic surgery on the hand	____________

Check your answers against the word and definition lists on the first page of this lesson. If you have any errors, count them and write the number in the blank at the top of the page. Practice any missed or misspelled words in the space provided. Sign your work and give it to your instructor. You may now go on to the next lesson.

PRACTICE

LESSON

7 Terminology Presentation

Listen to the Lab Tape provided by your instructor, and you will hear the words presented in this lesson. Read the words as they are said, noticing spelling and pronunciation. The recording will tell you when the presentation for this lesson is completed and will give you any further instructions. Do not go on to the next recorded lesson until you have completed Lesson 7 and feel that you know the words and word parts that have been presented.

• • • ▶ *Start Audio*

syndesm(o) a word element denoting ligaments

WORD	WORD PART	DEFINITION	ANSWER
1. syndesmectopia (sin′des-mek-to′pe-ah)	-ectopia	out of place	1. ________
2. syndesmorrhaphy (sin′des-mor′ah-fe)	-(o)rrhaphy	suture, surgical repair	2. ________
3. syndesmopexy (sin-des′mo-pek′se)	-pexy	fix, fasten	3. ________
4. syndesmitis (sin′des-mi′tis)	-itis	inflammation	4. ________
5. syndesmoplasty (sin-des′mo-plas′te)	-plasty	plastic surgery	5. ________
6. syndesmotomy (sin′des-mot′o-me)	-(o)tomy	incision, cutting into	6. ________
7. syndesmoma (sin′des-mo′mah)	-oma	tumor	7. ________

arthr(o) a word element denoting the joints

WORD	WORD PART	DEFINITION	ANSWER
8. arthrodysplasia (ar′thro-dis-pla′ze-ah)	dys -plasia	abnormal, painful formation	8. ________
9. arthralgia (ar-thral′je-ah)	-algia	pain	9. ________

10. arthritis (ar-thri'tis)	-itis	inflammation	10. ____________
11. arthroscope (ar'thro-skop)	-scope	viewing instrument	11. ____________
12. arthrocentesis (ar'thro-sen-te'sis)	-centesis	surgical puncture	12. ____________
13. arthrolith (ar'thro-lith)	-lith	stone	13. ____________
14. arthrodesis (ar'thro-de'sis)	-desis	binding, fixation	14. ____________
15. arthropathy (ar-throp'ah-the)	-pathy	disease	15. ____________
16. arthrosynovitis (ar'thro-sin'o-vi'tis)	synov(i) -itis	synovial membrane inflammation	16. ____________
17. arthrophyma (ar'thro-fi'mah)	-phyma	tumor, swelling	17. ____________

■ • • • *Stop Audio at Tone*

Study the 17 words and word parts for this lesson. Practice each word several times, checking your spelling and repeating the meaning to yourself. Listen to the recording and pronounce the words as many times as necessary. When you feel that you know the words and word parts well, you are ready to go on to the next step.

Use a sheet of paper to cover all columns except the Answer Column on the previous page. The words you have learned will be presented again on the recording. As each word is pronounced, write it in the space provided in the Answer Column.

• • • ▸ *Start Audio*

After stopping the tape player, check the words you have written against the words in the left-hand column. If any words are misspelled, practice writing them correctly. When you feel that you know and understand the words and word parts, go on to the Terminology Practice.

PRACTICE

____

____

____

____

____

Name ______________________ Date ______________ Errors ________

LESSON 7: TERMINOLOGY PRACTICE

Without looking at your previous work, write the word that is described by each definition.

syndesm(o) and *arthr(o)*

DEFINITION	TERM
1. Surgical fixation of a joint	______________
2. Any disease affecting a joint	______________
3. Suture or repair of ligaments	______________
4. Inflammation of a ligament	______________
5. Operative fixation of a dislocation using the joint ligaments	______________
6. Inflammation of a joint	______________
7. Surgical puncture and aspiration of a joint	______________
8. Swelling of a joint	______________
9. A connective tissue (ligament) tumor	______________
10. Displacement of a ligament	______________
11. Inflammation of the synovial membrane of a joint	______________
12. Pain in a joint	______________
13. An endoscope for examining the interior of a joint	______________
14. Plastic surgery on a ligament	______________
15. A calculous deposit in a joint	______________
16. The cutting of a ligament	______________
17. Abnormal joint development	______________

Check your answers against the word and definition lists on the first page of this lesson. If you have any errors, count them and write the number in the blank at the top of the page. Practice any missed or misspelled words in the space provided. Sign your work and give it to your instructor. You may now go on to the next lesson.

PRACTICE

LESSON 8

Terminology Presentation

Listen to the Lab Tape provided by your instructor, and you will hear the words presented in this lesson. Read the words as they are said, noticing spelling and pronunciation. The recording will tell you when the presentation for this lesson is completed and will give you any further instructions. Do not go on to the next recorded lesson until you have completed Lesson 8 and feel that you know the words and word parts that have been presented.

• • • ▶ *Start Audio*

spondyl(o) a word element indicating the vertebra or spinal column

WORD	WORD PART	DEFINITION	ANSWER
1. spondylopyosis (spon′di-lo-pi-o′sis)	py(o) -osis	pus, suppuration condition, process, increase, disease	1. ____________
2. spondylitis (spon′di-li′tis)	-itis	inflammation	2. ____________
3. spondylolisthesis (spon′di-lo-lis′the-sis)	-listhesis	to slip	3. ____________
4. spondylotherapy (spon′di-lo-ther′ah-pe)	-therapy	treatment	4. ____________
5. spondylomalacia (spon′di-lo-mah-la′she-ah)	-malacia	softening	5. ____________
6. spondylexarthrosis (spon′dil-eks′ar-thro′sis)	ex arthr(o) -osis	out joint condition, process, increase, disease	6. ____________
7. spondylalgia (spon′di-lal′je-ah)	-algia	pain	7. ____________

ten(o), tend(o) a word part denoting a tendon

WORD	WORD PART	DEFINITION	ANSWER
8. tendoplasty (ten′do-plas′te)	-plasty	plastic surgery	8. ____________
9. tenorrhaphy (ten-or′ah-fe)	-rrhaphy	suture, surgical repair	9. ____________

10. tenonectomy (ten′o-nek′to-me)	-ectomy	excision, removal	**10.** ______
11. tenodynia (ten′o-din′e-ah)	-dynia	pain	**11.** ______
12. tenotomy (ten-ot′o-me)	-tomy	incision, cutting into	**12.** ______
13. tenosynovitis (ten′o-sin′o-vi′tis)	synov(i) -itis	synovial membrane inflammation	**13.** ______
14. tenodesis (ten-od′e-sis)	-desis	binding, fixation	**14.** ______

■ • • • *Stop Audio at Tone*

Study the 14 words and word parts for this lesson. Practice each word several times, checking your spelling and repeating the meaning to yourself. Listen to the recording and pronounce the words as many times as necessary. When you feel that you know the words and word parts well, you are ready to go on to the next step.

Use a sheet of paper to cover all columns except the Answer Column on the previous page. The words you have learned will be presented again on the recording. As each word is pronounced, write it in the space provided in the Answer Column.

• • • ▸ *Start Audio*

After stopping the tape player, check the words you have written against the words in the left-hand column. If any words are misspelled, practice writing them correctly. When you feel that you know and understand the words and word parts, go on to the Terminology Practice.

PRACTICE

______

______

______

______

______

______

______

______

______

Name ______________________ Date ______________ Errors ________

LESSON 8: TERMINOLOGY PRACTICE

Without looking at your previous work, write the word that is described by each definition.

spondyl(o) and *ten(o), tend(o)*

DEFINITION	TERM
1. Treatment applied to the spinal region	______________
2. The union of a divided tendon by suture	______________
3. Excision of part of a tendon	______________
4. Inflammation of a tendon together with its sheath	______________
5. Pain in a vertebra	______________
6. Plastic surgery on a tendon	______________
7. Suppuration of one or more of the vertebral bodies	______________
8. Inflammation of a vertebra	______________
9. Tendon fixation	______________
10. The cutting of a tendon as for strabismus or clubfoot	______________
11. Slipping of one vertebra over another	______________
12. Pain in a tendon	______________
13. Softening of the vertebra	______________
14. A condition in which a vertebra is out of its joint or is dislocated	______________

Check your answers against the word and definition lists on the first page of this lesson. If you have any errors, count them and write the number in the blank at the top of the page. Practice any missed or misspelled words in the space provided. Sign your work and give it to your instructor. You may now go on to the next lesson.

PRACTICE

LESSON

9 Terminology Presentation

Listen to the Lab Tape provided by your instructor, and you will hear the words presented in this lesson. Read the words as they are said, noticing spelling and pronunciation. The recording will tell you when the presentation for this lesson is completed and will give you any further instructions. Do not go on to the next recorded lesson until you have completed Lesson 9 and feel that you know the words and word parts that have been presented.

Start Audio

chondr(o) a word part denoting cartilage

WORD	WORD PART	DEFINITION	ANSWER
1. chondrodysplasia (kon′dro-dis-pla′ze-ah)	dys -plasia	abnormal, painful formation	1. ________
2. chondrophyte (kon′dro-fit)	-phytos	a growth	2. ________
3. chondrolipoma (kon′dro-lip-o′mah)	lip(o) -oma	fat tumor	3. ________
4. chondrolysis (kon-drol′i-sis)	-lysis	dissolve, break down	4. ________
5. chondritis (kon-dri′tis)	-itis	inflammation	5. ________
6. chondrocostal (kon-dro-kos′tal)	cost -al	rib of, pertaining to	6. ________
7. chondropathy (kon-drop′ah-the)	-pathy	disease	7. ________

my(o) a word element denoting muscle

WORD	WORD PART	DEFINITION	ANSWER
8. myasthenia (mi′as-the′ne-ah)	a- -sthenia	without, lack of strength	8. ________
9. myorrhexis (mi′o-rek′sis)	-rrhexis	rupture	9. ________
10. myocardial (mi′o-kar′de-al)	card(i) -al	heart of, pertaining to	10. ________

11. myokinesis (mi′o-ki-ne′sis)	-kinesis	movement	11. ________
12. myoplasty (mi′o-plas′te)	-plasty	plastic surgery	12. ________
13. myodynia (mi′o-din′e-ah)	-dynia	pain	13. ________
14. myotasis (mi-ot′ah-sis)	-tasis	stretching	14. ________
15. myoblastoma (mi′o-blas-to′mah)	blast -oma	immature cell tumor	15. ________
16. myocardiopathy (mi′o-kar′de-op′ah-the)	cardi(o) -pathy	heart disease	16. ________
17. myomalacia (mi′o-mah-la′she-ah)	-malacia	softening	17. ________

■ • • • *Stop Audio at Tone*

Study the 17 words and word parts for this lesson. Practice each word several times, checking your spelling and repeating the meaning to yourself. Listen to the recording and pronounce the words as many times as necessary. When you feel that you know the words and word parts well, you are ready to go on to the next step.

Use a sheet of paper to cover all columns except the Answer Column on the previous page. The words you have learned will be presented again on the recording. As each word is pronounced, write it in the space provided in the Answer Column.

• • • ▶ *Start Audio*

After stopping the tape player, check the words you have written against the words in the left-hand column. If any words are misspelled, practice writing them correctly. When you feel that you know and understand the words and word parts, go on to the Terminology Practice.

PRACTICE

____

____

____

____

____

____

Name ______________________ Date ______________ Errors ________

LESSON 9: TERMINOLOGY PRACTICE

Without looking at your previous work, write the word that is described by each definition.

chondr(o) and *my(o)*

DEFINITION	TERM
1. Movement of muscles	______________
2. Plastic surgery on a muscle	______________
3. A cartilaginous growth at the articular extremity of a bone	______________
4. Pertaining to the muscular tissue of the heart	______________
5. Stretching of a muscle	______________
6. Abnormal formation of cartilage	______________
7. A cartilaginous and fatty tissue tumor	______________
8. Weakness of a muscle	______________
9. Degeneration of cartilage	______________
10. Of or pertaining to the ribs and costal cartilages	______________
11. Softening of the muscles	______________
12. A disease of the heart muscle	______________
13. Muscle pain	______________
14. A tumor of immature muscle cells	______________
15. A disease of cartilage	______________
16. Rupture or tearing of a muscle	______________
17. Inflammation of cartilage	______________

Check your answers against the word and definition lists on the first page of this lesson. If you have any errors, count them and write the number in the blank at the top of the page. Practice any missed or misspelled words in the space provided. Sign your work and give it to your instructor. You may now go on to the next lesson.

PRACTICE

Name ______________________ Date ______________ Errors ________

LESSON 10 — TERMINOLOGY REVIEW FOR TEST 2

This is a review of the word parts you have learned in the preceding four lessons. Some of the terms to be listed below may be new, but they are made up of word parts that you have already learned.

Unlike the review for Test 1, the words are not written out for you. As each word is pronounced on the Lab Tape, write it in the appropriate numbered blank on the left.

• • • ▸ *Start Audio*

WORD	WORD PART	MEANING OF WORD PART
1. ______	______	______
	______	______
	______	______
2. ______	______	______
	______	______
	______	______
3. ______	______	______
	______	______
	______	______
4. ______	______	______
	______	______
	______	______
5. ______	______	______
	______	______
	______	______
6. ______	______	______
	______	______
	______	______
7. ______	______	______
	______	______
	______	______
8. ______	______	______
	______	______
	______	______

9. ______________________ ______________ ____________________________________

______________ ____________________________________

______________ ____________________________________

10. ______________________ ______________ ____________________________________

______________ ____________________________________

______________ ____________________________________

11. ______________________ ______________ ____________________________________

______________ ____________________________________

______________ ____________________________________

12. ______________________ ______________ ____________________________________

______________ ____________________________________

______________ ____________________________________

13. ______________________ ______________ ____________________________________

______________ ____________________________________

______________ ____________________________________

14. ______________________ ______________ ____________________________________

______________ ____________________________________

______________ ____________________________________

15. ______________________ ______________ ____________________________________

______________ ____________________________________

______________ ____________________________________

■ • • • *Stop Audio at Tone*

After all 15 words have been written, write the word parts for each one and fill in the meanings of the parts. Use the Glossary or a dictionary to check your spellings and definitions. Practice the words on a separate sheet of paper, paying particular attention to any you missed or misspelled.

When you feel you know the words and word parts well, sign your work, indicate the number of errors, and turn your work in to your instructor.

You are now ready for the Extra Credit Review (if your instructor assigns it) or Test 2.

Name ______________________ Date ______________ Errors ________

LESSON 10 | **EXTRA CREDIT REVIEW**

This Extra Credit Review should be done at the discretion of your instructor. If you are instructed to complete this portion of the Review, turn it in to your instructor when you are finished.

PART A

Each phrase below defines one of the words you have just studied. Without looking at your previous work, fill in the word that matches each definition.

DEFINITION	TERM
1. Softening of a bone	______________
2. A calculous deposit in a joint	______________
3. A tumor of immature muscle cells	______________
4. Suppuration of one or more of the vertebral bodies	______________
5. Displacement of a ligament	______________
6. Pain in the hands and feet	______________
7. Inflammation of a bone	______________
8. Plastic surgery on a muscle	______________
9. Abnormal formation of cartilage	______________
10. Tendon fixation	______________
11. Suture or repair of ligaments	______________
12. Pain in a joint	______________
13. Enlargement of the hands	______________
14. A condition in which a vertebra is out of its joint or is dislocated	______________
15. The cutting of a tendon as for strabismus or clubfoot	______________

PART B

Match the following terms with the definitions given. Place the correct letter of the term to the left of the definition.

DEFINITION

_______ **16.** A connective tissue (ligament) tumor

_______ **17.** Pain in a tendon

_______ **18.** A condition in which a vertebra is out of its joint or is dislocated

_______ **19.** A cartilaginous growth at the articular extremity of a bone

_______ **20.** Pain in the hands or feet

_______ **21.** A tumor of immature muscle cells

_______ **22.** Reduction in the quantity of bone or atrophy of skeletal tissues

_______ **23.** Movement of the muscles

_______ **24.** An endoscope for the examination of the interior of a joint

_______ **25.** A calculous deposit in a joint

TERM

a. cheiropodalgia
b. osteoporosis
c. arthroscope
d. syndesmoma
e. spondylexarthrosis
f. arthrolith
g. chondrophyte
h. tenodynia
i. myoblastoma
j. myokinesis

You may now go on to Test 2.

SECTION 3

Integumentary System

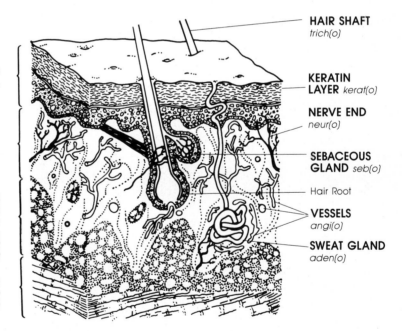

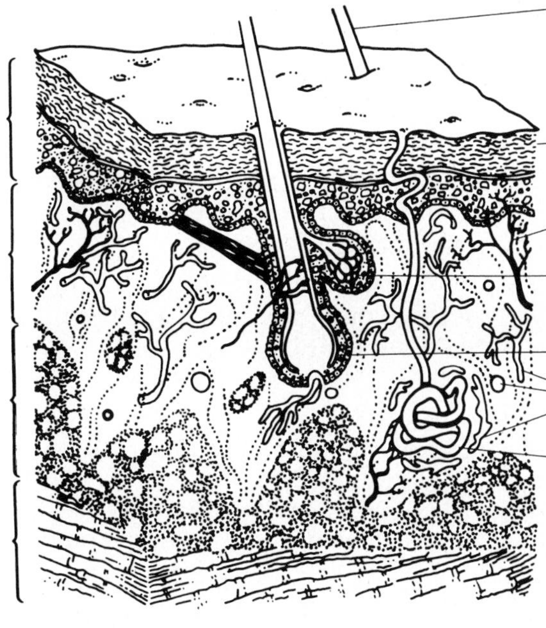

INTEGUMENTARY SYSTEM

Orientation

The integumentary system consists of the skin, nails, hair, and glands embedded in the skin. The skin (integument) has been called the largest organ of the body because of its great surface area. The skin provides a protective covering, acts as a sensing unit to note changes in the environment, and helps to regulate body temperature.

The skin consists of three layers: the epidermis, the dermis, and the subcutaneous tissue. The epidermis is a protective covering of scalelike cells made up of the protein keratin. It sheds water, prevents evaporation of body fluids, and keeps germs from entering the deeper layers. The epidermis has several layers. The outermost layer, stratum corneum, is composed of flat, horny cells which are shed constantly. New cells are pushed forward from deeper layers of the epidermis. Color in the epidermis is the result of pigment granules called melanin. This pigment protects the body from excess ultraviolet light rays. It also gives rise to differences in color between the races. Fingerprints are formed by ridges in the epidermis.

The dermis, also called the corium, contains the hair follicles (roots), sebaceous (oil) glands, sudoriferous (sweat) glands, and sense receptors that signal the brain when they feel pain, heat, cold, or pressure. The body has some two million sweat glands. There are two kinds of sudoriferous or sweat glands, apocrine and eccrine. Apocrine glands are found in the pubic, anal, and mammary regions. Eccrine glands are found almost everywhere in the body and help the body to handle excessive heat.

The subcutaneous layer of the skin is a combination of fibrous and fatty tissues. The fibrous tissue attaches the upper skin layers to the skeletal muscles. The fatty tissue holds in body heat and acts as an insulator against cold.

Hair and nails are forms of skin cells. Keratin is the major structure of this tissue. Nails are made up of the same materials as hair, but they are hard, flat plates.

LESSON 11

Terminology Presentation

Listen to the Lab Tape provided by your instructor, and you will hear the words presented in this lesson. Read the words as they are said, noticing spelling and pronunciation. The recording will tell you when the presentation for this lesson is completed and will give you any further instructions. Do not go on to the next recorded lesson until you have completed Lesson 11 and feel that you know the words and word parts that have been presented.

• • • ▸ *Start Audio*

kerat(o) a combining form denoting the cornea of the eye or horny tissue

WORD	WORD PART	DEFINITION	ANSWER
1. keratiasis (ker′ah-ti′ah-sis)	-iasis	diseased condition	1. ________
2. keratoderma (ker′ah-to-der′mah)	derm(a)	skin	2. ________
3. keratoid (ker′ah-toid)	-oid	like, resembling	3. ________
4. keratogenous (ker′ah-toj′e-nus)	-genous	to produce	4. ________
5. keratoma (ker′ah-to′mah)	-oma	tumor	5. ________

derm(o), derm(a), or ***dermat(o)*** a word element denoting the skin

WORD	WORD PART	DEFINITION	ANSWER
6. dermatologist (der′mah-tol′o-jist)	-(o)logist	specialist	6. ________
7. dermatoautoplasty (der′mah-to-aw′to-plas′te)	auto -plasty	self plastic surgery	7. ________
8. dermatitis (der′mah-ti′tis)	-itis	inflammation	8. ________

9. dermatoconiosis (der'mah-to-ko-ne-o'sis)	coni(o) -osis	dust condition, process, increase, disease	9. ______
10. dermal (der'mal)	-al	of, pertaining to	10. ______
11. dermatophobia (der'mah-to-fo'be-ah)	-phobia	fear	11. ______
12. dermatosis (der'mah-to'sis)	-osis	condition, process, increase, disease	12. ______
13. dermatome (der'mah-tom)	-tome	an instrument for cutting	13. ______
14. dermomycosis (der'mo-mi-ko'sis)	mycosis	fungus	14. ______
15. dermatorrhea (der'mah-to-re'ah)	-rrhea	flow	15. ______

■ • • • *Stop Audio at Tone*

Study the 15 words and word parts for this lesson. Practice each word several times, checking your spelling and repeating the meaning to yourself. Listen to the recording and pronounce the words as many times as necessary. When you feel that you know the words and word parts well, you are ready to go on to the next step.

Use a sheet of paper to cover all columns except the Answer Column on the previous page. The words you have learned will be presented again on the recording. As each word is pronounced, write it in the space provided in the Answer Column.

• • • ▶ *Start Audio*

After stopping the tape player, check the words you have written against the words in the left-hand column. If any words are misspelled, practice writing them correctly. When you feel that you know and understand the words and word parts, go on to the Terminology Practice.

PRACTICE

______

______

______

______

______

______

Name ______________________ Date ______________ Errors ________

LESSON 11: TERMINOLOGY PRACTICE

Without looking at your previous work, write the word that is described by each definition.

kerat(o) and *derm(o) derm(a), dermat(o)*

DEFINITION	TERM
1. Of or pertaining to the skin	________
2. Autografting of skin taken from another part of the patient's own body	________
3. A horny skin or covering	________
4. The presence of horny warts on the skin	________
5. An instrument for cutting the skin or cutting thin transplants	________
6. Specialist in the diagnosis and treatment of skin diseases	________
7. Any fungus disease of the skin	________
8. A morbid fear of acquiring a skin disease	________
9. A tumor or growth of horny tissue	________
10. Producing cells that result in the formation of horny tissue such as fingernails	________
11. Any generalized skin disease	________
12. An occupational dermatitis caused by irritation by dust	________
13. Inflammation of the skin	________
14. An excessive secretion of the sebaceous or sweat glands of the skin	________
15. Like or resembling a horny skin	________

Check your answers against the word and definition lists on the first page of this lesson. If you have any errors, count them and write the number in the blank at the top of the page. Practice any missed or misspelled words on the next page. Sign your work and give it to your instructor. You are now ready for the next lesson.

PRACTICE

LESSON

12

Terminology Presentation

Listen to the Lab Tape provided by your instructor, and you will hear the words presented in this lesson. Read the words as they are said, noticing spelling and pronunciation. The recording will tell you when the presentation for this lesson is completed and will give you any further instructions. Do not go on to the next recorded lesson until you have completed Lesson 12 and feel that you know the words and word parts that have been presented.

• • • ▶ *Start Audio*

trich, trich(o) a word part indicating the hair or the capillary (hairlike) vessels

WORD	WORD PART	DEFINITION	ANSWER
1. trichoglossia (trik'o-glos'e-ah)	-gloss	pertaining to the tongue	1. ______
2. trichalgia (trik-al'je-ah)	-algia	pain	2. ______
3. trichoclasis (trik-ok'lah-sis)	-clasis	break, fracture	3. ______
4. trichoschisis (trik-os'ki-sis)	-schisis	splitting	4. ______
5. trichopathy (tri-kop'ah-the)	-pathy	disease	5. ______
6. trichomycosis (trik'o-mi-ko'sis)	-myc(o) -osis	fungus condition, process, increase, disease	6. ______
7. trichogenous (tri-koj'e-nus)	-genous	to produce	7. ______

hist(o), histi(o) a word part denoting relationship to tissue

WORD	WORD PART	DEFINITION	ANSWER
8. histology (his-tol'o-je)	-(o)logy	study of, science of	8. ______
9. histanoxia (his'tan-ok'se-ah)	an -oxia	without, lack of oxygen	9. ______

10. histoneurology (his'to-nu-rol'o-je)	neur(o) -(o)logy	nerves study of, science of	10. ______
11. histokinesis (his'to-ki-ne'sis)	-kinesis	movement	11. ______
12. histocyte (his'to-sit)	-cyte	cell	12. ______
13. histotoxic (his'to-tok'sik)	tox -ic	poison pertaining to	13. ______
14. historrhexis (his'to-rek'sis)	-rrhexis	rupture	14. ______

■ • • • *Stop Audio at Tone*

Study the 14 words and word parts for this lesson. Practice each word several times, checking your spelling and repeating the meaning to yourself. Listen to the recording and pronounce the words as many times as necessary. When you feel that you know the words and word parts well, you are ready to go on to the next step.

Use a sheet of paper to cover all columns except the Answer Column on the previous page. The words you have learned will be presented again on the recording. As each word is pronounced, write it in the space provided in the Answer Column.

• • • ▸ *Start Audio*

After stopping the tape player, check the words you have written against the words in the left-hand column. If any words are misspelled, practice writing them correctly. When you feel that you know and understand the words and word parts, go on to the Terminology Practice.

PRACTICE

Name ______________________________ Date __________________ Errors ________

LESSON 12: TERMINOLOGY PRACTICE

Without looking at your previous work, write the word that is described by each definition.

trich(o) or *hist(o), histi(o)*

DEFINITION	TERM
1. A hairy condition of the tongue	______________
2. The histology of the nervous system	______________
3. Oxygen deprivation of tissue, usually resulting from lack of blood supply	______________
4. Pain when the hair is touched	______________
5. A tissue cell	______________
6. Promoting growth of hair	______________
7. Splitting of the hair	______________
8. The study of tissue	______________
9. Abnormal brittleness of the hair	______________
10. Breaking up of tissue	______________
11. A disease of the hair	______________
12. Being poisonous to tissue or tissues	______________
13. Movement in the tissues of the body	______________
14. Fungus infection of the hair	______________

Check your answers against the word and definition lists on the first page of this lesson. If you have any errors, count them and write the number in the blank at the top of the page. Practice any missed or misspelled words on the next page. Sign your work and give it to your instructor. You are now ready for the next lesson.

PRACTICE

LESSON 13

Terminology Presentation

Listen to the Lab Tape provided by your instructor, and you will hear the words presented in this lesson. Read the words as they are said, noticing spelling and pronunciation. The recording will tell you when the presentation for this lesson is completed and will give you any further instructions. Do not go on to the next recorded lesson until you have completed Lesson 13.

••• ▶ *Start Audio*

sarc(o) a word element denoting flesh or connective tissue

WORD	WORD PART	DEFINITION	ANSWER
1. sarcopoietic (sar′ko-poi-et′ik)	-poiet -ic	to make, produce pertaining to	1. ______
2. sarcoid (sar′koid)	-oid	like, resembling	2. ______
3. sarcolysis (sar-kol′i-sis)	-(o)lysis	dissolve, break down	3. ______
4. sarcomphalocele (sar′kom-fal′o-sel)	omphal(o) -cele	navel, umbilicus tumor, swelling, hernia	4. ______
5. sarcoma (sar-ko′mah)	-oma	tumor	5. ______
6. sarcosepsis (sar′ko-sep′sis)	-sepsis	poison	6. ______
7. sarcoblast (sar′ko-blast)	-blast	immature cell	7. ______
8. sarcostosis (sar′kos-to′sis)	-ost(eo) -osis	bone condition, process, increase, disease	8. ______

onych(o) a word element denoting the nails

WORD	WORD PART	DEFINITION	ANSWER
9. onychomalacia (on′i-ko-mah-la′she-ah)	-malacia	softening	9. ______

10. onychophagia (on′i-ko-fa′je-ah)	-phagia	to eat	**10.** ______________
11. onychorrhexis (on′i-ko-rek′sis)	-rrhexis	rupture	**11.** ______________
12. onychoma (on′i-ko′mah)	-oma	tumor	**12.** ______________
13. onychomycosis (on′i-ko-mi-ko′sis)	-myc(o) -osis	fungus condition, process, increase, disease	**13.** ______________
14. onychosis (on′i-ko′sis)	-osis	condition, process, increase, disease	**14.** ______________
15. onychoptosis (on′i-kop-to′sis)	-ptosis	falling	**15.** ______________
16. onychogenic (on′i-ko-jen′ik)	-genic	produce	**16.** ______________

■ • • • *Stop Audio at Tone*

Study the 16 words and word parts for this lesson. Practice each word several times, checking your spelling and repeating the meaning to yourself. Listen to the recording and pronounce the words as many times as necessary. When you feel that you know the words and word parts well, you are ready to go on to the next step.

Use a sheet of paper to cover all columns except the Answer Column on the previous page. The words you have learned will be presented again on the recording. As each word is pronounced, write it in the space provided in the Answer Column.

• • • ▸ *Start Audio*

After stopping the tape player, check the words you have written against the words in the left-hand column. If any words are misspelled, practice writing them correctly. When you feel that you know and understand the words and word parts, go on to the Terminology Practice.

PRACTICE

____

____

____

____

____

____

Name ______________________________ Date ____________________ Errors __________

LESSON 13: TERMINOLOGY PRACTICE

Without looking at your previous work, write the word that is described by each definition.

sarc(o) and *onych(o)*

DEFINITION	TERM
1. Tumor of fleshy or connective tissue	______________
2. Softening of the fingernail	______________
3. Producing nail substance	______________
4. Falling off of the nail	______________
5. Habitual biting of the nails	______________
6. Destruction or dissolution of flesh	______________
7. A fleshy tumor of the umbilicus	______________
8. Ossification of the fleshy tissues	______________
9. A disease of the nails	______________
10. A tumor of the nail or nail bed	______________
11. Fungus condition of the nails	______________
12. Producing flesh or muscle	______________
13. Like or resembling flesh	______________
14. Primitive or immature cell which develops into connective tissue	______________
15. Sepsis due to the presence of bacteria in the tissues	______________
16. Splitting or rupture of the nails	______________

Check your answers against the word and definition lists on the first page of this lesson. If you have any errors, count them and write the number in the blank at the top of the page. Practice any missed or misspelled words on the next page. Sign your work and give it to your instructor. You are now ready for the next lesson.

PRACTICE

LESSON 14

Terminology Presentation

Listen to the Lab Tape provided by your instructor, and you will hear the words presented in this lesson. Read the words as they are said, noticing spelling and pronunciation. The recording will tell you when the presentation for this lesson is completed and will give you any further instructions. Do not go on to the next recorded lesson until you have completed Lesson 14 and feel that you know the words and word parts that have been presented.

• • • ▸ *Start Audio*

cheil(o) a combining form denoting relationship to the lip

WORD	WORD PART	DEFINITION	ANSWER
1. cheilitis (ki-li'tis)	-itis	inflammation	1. ________
2. cheilophagia (ki'lo-fa'je-ah)	-phagia	to eat	2. ________
3. cheilostomatoplasty (ki'lo-sto-mat'o-plas'te)	stomat(o) -plasty	mouth plastic surgery	3. ________
4. cheilotomy (ki-lot'o-me)	-tomy	incision, cutting into	4. ________
5. cheilocarcinoma (ki'lo-kar'si-no'mah)	-carcinoma	cancer	5. ________
6. cheiloschisis (ki-los'ki-sis)	-schisis	splitting	6. ________
7. cheilorrhaphy (ki-lor'ah-fe)	-rrhaphy	suture, surgical repair	7. ________
8. cheilectomy (ki-lek'to-me)	-ectomy	excision, removal	8. ________

mast(o) a combining form denoting relationship to the breast or mammary gland

WORD	WORD PART	DEFINITION	ANSWER
9. mastitis (mas-ti'tis)	-itis	inflammation	9. ________

10. mastodynia (mas'to-din'e-ah)	-dynia	pain	10. ________
11. mastosis (mas-to'sis)	-osis	condition, process, increase, disease	11. ________
12. mastopexy (mas'to-pek-se)	-pexy	fix, fasten	12. ________
13. mastectomy (mas-tek'to-me)	-ectomy	excision, removal	13. ________
14. mastoplasty (mas'to-plas'te)	-plasty	plastic surgery	14. ________
15. mastoid (mas'toid)	-oid	like, resembling	15. ________
16. mastoscirrhus (mas'to-skir'us)	-scirrhus	hardening	16. ________

■ • • • *Stop Audio at Tone*

Study the 16 words and word parts for this lesson. Practice each word several times, checking your spelling and repeating the meaning to yourself. Listen to the recording and pronounce the words as many times as necessary. When you feel that you know the words and word parts well, you are ready to go on to the next step.

Use a sheet of paper to cover all columns except the Answer Column on the previous page. The words you have learned will be presented again on the recording. As each word is pronounced, write it in the space provided in the Answer Column.

• • • ▸ *Start Audio*

After stopping the tape player, check the words you have written against the words in the left-hand column. If any words are misspelled, practice writing them correctly. When you feel that you know and understand the words and word parts, go on to the Terminology Practice.

PRACTICE

Name ______________________ Date ________________ Errors __________

LESSON 14: TERMINOLOGY PRACTICE

Without looking at your previous work, write the word that is described by each definition.

cheil(o) and *mast(o)*

DEFINITION	TERM
1. Excision of the breast	______________
2. Cleft in the lip, harelip	______________
3. Surgical fixation of a pendulous or sagging breast	______________
4. Inflammation of the lip	______________
5. Resembling a nipple or breast	______________
6. Any disease of the breast	______________
7. Plastic surgery on the lip and mouth	______________
8. Pain in a breast	______________
9. Habitual biting of the lip	______________
10. Excision of the lip as for cheilocarcinoma	______________
11. Hardening of the mammary gland	______________
12. Incision into the lip	______________
13. Cancer of the lip	______________
14. Plastic surgery on the breast	______________
15. Inflammation of the breast	______________
16. Suture of the lip	______________

Check your answers against the word and definition lists on the first page of this lesson. If you have any errors, count them and write the number in the blank at the top of the page. Practice any missed or misspelled words on the next page. Sign your work and give it to your instructor. You are now ready for the next lesson.

PRACTICE

Name ______________________ Date ______________ Errors ________

LESSON 15 | TERMINOLOGY REVIEW FOR TEST 3

This is a review of the word parts you have learned in the preceding four lessons. Some of the medical terms listed below may be new, but they are made up of word parts that you have already learned. Read the words below as they are pronounced on the Lab Tape. As you listen, notice the familiar word parts which make them up.

• • • ▸ *Start Audio*

WORD	WORD PART	MEANING OF WORD PART
1. histocyte	hist(o)	________
(his′to-sit)	-cyte	________
histocyte	________	________
2. dermomycosis	derm(o)	________
(der′mo-mi-ko′sis)	-mycosis	________
dermomycosis	________	________
3. trichalgia	trich(o)	________
(trik-al′je-ah)	-algia	________
trichalgia	________	________
4. keratoma	kerat(o)	________
(ker′ah-to′mah)	-oma	________
keratoma	________	________
5. sarcolysis	sarc(o)	________
(sar-kol′i-sis)	-(o)lysis	________
sarcolysis	________	________
6. onychophagia	onych(o)	________
(on′i-ko-fa′je-ah)	-phagia	________
onychophagia	________	________
7. mastoscirrhus	mast(o)	________
(mas′to-skir′us)	-scirrhus	________
mastoscirrhus	________	________
8. cheilophagia	cheil(o)	________
(ki′lo-fa′je-ah)	-phagia	________
cheilophagia	________	________

9. histology — hist(o) ____________________
(his-tol′o-je) — -(o)logy ____________________
histology ______________________________________

10. dermatitis — dermat ____________________
(der′mah-ti′tis) — -itis ____________________
dermatitis ______________________________________

11. histotoxic — hist(o) ____________________
(his′to-tok′sik) — tox ____________________
-ic ____________________
histotoxic ______________________________________

12. sarcosepsis — sarc(o) ____________________
(sar-ko-sep′sis) — -sepsis ____________________
sarcosepsis ______________________________________

13. onychomalacia — onych(o) ____________________
(on′i-ko-mah-la′she-ah) — -malacia ____________________
onychomalacia ______________________________________

14. cheilocarcinoma — cheil(o) ____________________
(ki′lo-kar′si-no′mah) — -carcinoma ____________________
cheilocarcinoma ______________________________________

15. mastopexy — mast(o) ____________________
(mas′to-pek-se) — -pexy ____________________
mastopexy ______________________________________

■ • • • *Stop Audio at Tone*

On the lines provided, fill in the meanings of as many of the word parts as you can from memory. Then, use the previous lessons or a medical dictionary to look up any definitions you could not remember. Fill them in. On a separate piece of paper, practice writing the word parts and their meanings. Pay special attention to any which you had trouble remembering. Be sure to check your spelling.

When you have defined and reviewed all the word parts, write a definition for each whole word on the line provided. Check your definitions in the Glossary or a medical dictionary and make any needed corrections. Practice the words on a separate sheet of paper until you are sure that you know them. Then go on to the Extra Credit Review (if your instructor assigns it) or Test 3.

Name ______________________ Date ______________ Errors ________

LESSON 15 — EXTRA CREDIT REVIEW

This Extra Credit Review should be done at the discretion of your instructor. If you are instructed to complete this portion of the Review, turn it into your instructor when you are finished.

PART A

Each phrase below defines one of the words you have just studied. Without looking at your previous work, fill in the word that matches each definition.

DEFINITION	TERM
1. Pain when the hair is touched	______________
2. Inflammation of the skin	______________
3. Being poisonous to tissue or tissues	______________
4. Habitual biting of the lip	______________
5. Any fungus disease of the skin	______________
6. Cancer of the lip	______________
7. The study of tissue	______________
8. Dissolution of flesh	______________
9. Surgical fixation of a pendulous or sagging breast	______________
10. A tissue cell	______________
11. Sepsis due to the presence of bacteria in the tissue	______________
12. A tumor or growth of horny tissue	______________
13. Hardening of the mammary gland	______________
14. Softening of the fingernail	______________
15. Habitual biting of the nails	______________

PART B

Match the following terms with the definitions given. Place the correct letter of the term to the left of the definition.

DEFINITION	TERM
______ 16. Producing cells that result in the formation of horny tissue such as a fingernail	a. cheiloschisis
______ 17. An occupational dermatitis caused by irritation by dust	b. mastectomy
______ 18. Splitting of the hair	c. histanoxia
______ 19. Cleft in the lip, harelip	d. onychomycosis
______ 20. A specialist in the diagnosis and treatment of skin diseases	e. keratogenous
______ 21. A fungus condition of the nails	f. sarcostosis
______ 22. Excision of the breast	g. trichoschisis
______ 23. A fleshy tumor of the umbilicus	h. dermatoconiosis
______ 24. Ossification of fleshy tissues	i. dermatologist
______ 25. Oxygen deprivation of tissue usually resulting from lack of blood supply	j. sarcomphalocele

You may now go on to Test 3.

SECTION

4 Genitourinary System

URINARY TRACT
ur(o)

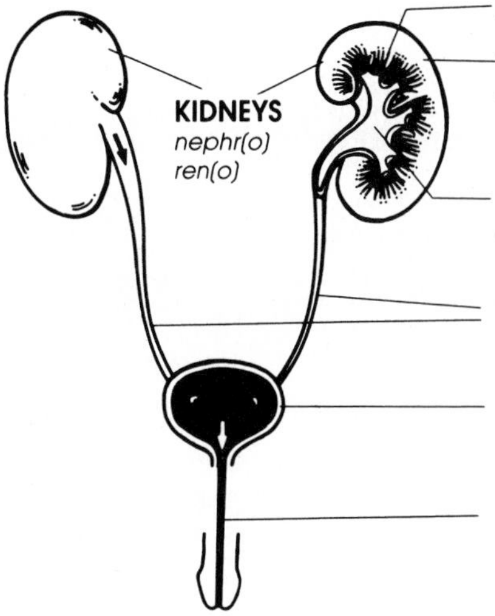

MALE GENITALIA
genit(o)

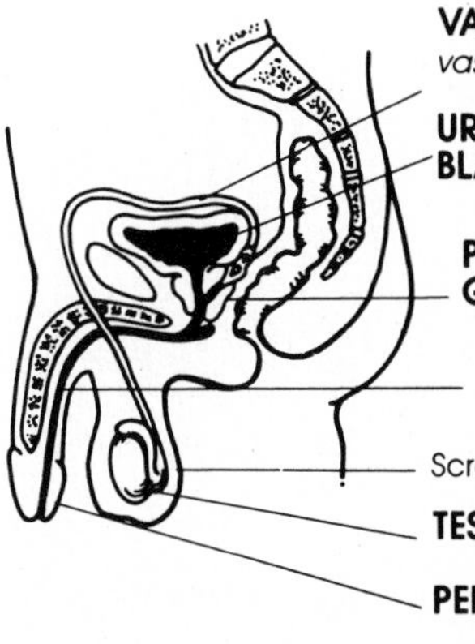

FEMALE GENITALIA

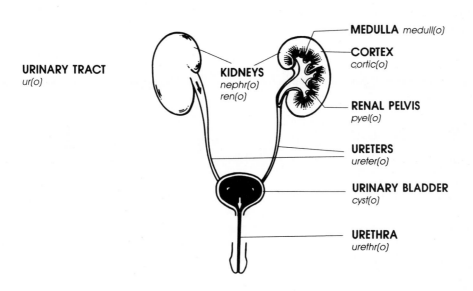

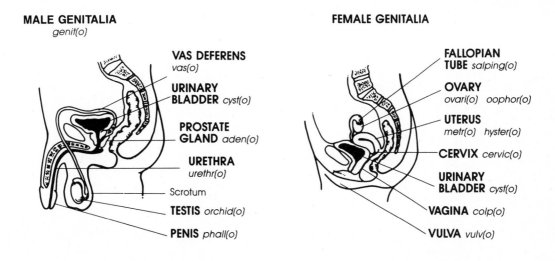

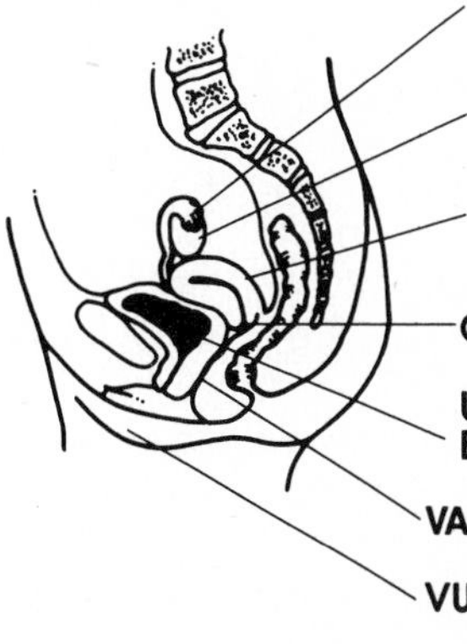

GENITOURINARY SYSTEM

Orientation

The genitourinary system is really two systems: the reproductive system, which consists of the male and female organs of reproduction (genitalia), and the urinary system, which contains the structures for excreting and removing fluid wastes from the body.

The internal female genitalia consist of two ovaries that produce the female sex cells (ovum), two uterine or fallopian tubes that convey the egg to the uterus (a pear-shaped organ designed to hold and nourish a developing fetus), and the vagina which provides access to the uterus. The external female genitalia, known as the vulva, include the mons pubis, the labia (lips) minora and majora, and the clitoris.

The male genitalia consist of the testes, epididymis, vas deferens, ejaculatory duct, urethra, and penis. The male testes are located outside the body. They are contained in a sac called the scrotum. The testes produce spermatozoa (sperm) and the male hormone, testosterone. This hormone causes body hair and the deepening of the male voice. Maturation of sperm takes place in the epididymis or spermatic cord. They then move on to the vas deferens (ductus deferens) which is a continuation of the epididymis. The vas deferens continues up to the interior surface of the urinary bladder where each segment of the vas deferens joins the duct of the seminal vesicles, which are two membranous pouches. The duct of each joins with the vas deferens to form the ejaculatory duct.

The urinary system is composed of two kidneys, two ureters, a urinary bladder, and the urethra. In the male, the prostate gland surrounds the first section of the urethra and secretes a substance which protects the sperm cells from the acidity of the vaginal secretions. The urinary system is responsible for excreting wastes from the blood, regulating the amount of water in the body, and keeping the pH (relation of acids to bases) in balance. The blood is filtered in the kidneys, where certain fluids and minerals are reabsorbed. The remaining fluid wastes are collected in the urinary bladder. They pass out of the body through the urethra during urination.

LESSON

16 Terminology Presentation

Listen to the Lab Tape provided by your instructor, and you will hear the words presented in this lesson. Read the words as they are said, noticing spelling and pronunciation. The recording will tell you when the presentation for this lesson is completed and will give you any further instructions. Do not go on to the next recorded lesson until you have completed Lesson 16 and feel that you know the words and word parts that have been presented.

• • • ▶ *Start Audio*

pyel(o) a word part denoting the pelvis of the kidney

WORD	WORD PART	DEFINITION	ANSWER
1. pyelography (pi′e-log′rah-fe)	-graphy	recording	1. ____
2. pyelitis (pi′e-li′tis)	-itis	inflammation	2. ____
3. pyeloscopy (pi′e-los′ko-pe)	-scopy	examine	3. ____
4. pyelocystitis (pi′e-lo-sis-ti′tis)	cyst -itis	urinary bladder inflammation	4. ____
5. pyelophlebitis (pi′e-lo-fle-bi′tis)	phleb(o) -itis	vein inflammation	5. ____
6. pyelectasis (pi′e-lek′tah-sis)	-ectasis	dilatation, expansion	6. ____
7. pyelolithotomy (pi′e-lo-li-thot′o-me)	lith -tomy	stone incision, cutting into	7. ____

uria a word ending or suffix having to do with the urine or urination

WORD	WORD PART	DEFINITION	ANSWER
8. melanuria (mel′an-u′re-ah)	melan(o)	black	8. ____

9. dysuria (dis-u′re-ah)	dys	abnormal, painful	9. ________
10. albuminuria (al′bu-mi-nu′re-ah)	albumin	white (protein)	10. ________
11. hematuria (hem′ah-tu′re-ah)	hemat(o)	blood	11. ________
12. polyuria (pol′e-u′re-ah)	poly	many	12. ________
13. nocturia (nok-tu′re-ah)	noct	night	13. ________
14. bacteriuria (bak-te′re-u′re-ah)	bacter(i)	bacteria	14. ________
15. pyuria (pi-u′re-ah)	py(o)	pus, suppuration	15. ________

■ • • • *Stop Audio at Tone*

Study the 15 words and word parts for this lesson. Practice each word several times, checking your spelling and repeating the meaning to yourself. Listen to the recording and pronounce the words as many times as necessary. When you feel that you know the words and word parts well, you are ready to go on to the next step.

Use a sheet of paper to cover all columns except the Answer Column on the previous page. The words you have learned will be presented again on the recording. As each word is pronounced, write it in the space provided in the Answer Column.

• • • ▶ *Start Audio*

After stopping the tape player, check the words you have written against the words in the left-hand column. If any words are misspelled, practice writing them correctly. When you feel that you know and understand the words and word parts, go on to the Terminology Practice.

PRACTICE

____

____

____

____

____

____

Name ______________________ Date ______________ Errors ________

LESSON 16: TERMINOLOGY PRACTICE

Without looking at your previous work, write the word that is described by each definition.

pyel(o) and *uria*

DEFINITION	TERM
1. Examination or observation of the kidney pelvis via a fluoroscope	____________
2. Black or dark discoloration of the urine	____________
3. Roentgenographic study of the kidney and renal collecting system	____________
4. Presence of pus in the urine	____________
5. Inflammation of the pelvis of the kidney	____________
6. Presence of bacteria in the urine	____________
7. Dilatation of the kidney pelvis	____________
8. Painful or difficult urination	____________
9. Excessive urination at night	____________
10. Inflammation of the renal pelvis and bladder	____________
11. Presence of blood in the urine	____________
12. The operation of removing a renal calculus from the pelvis of the kidney	____________
13. Inflammation of the veins of the renal pelvis	____________
14. Presence of serum albumin in the urine	____________
15. Excessive excretion of urine	____________

Check your answers against the word and definition lists on the first page of this lesson. If you have any errors, count them and write the number in the blank at the top of the page. Practice any missed or misspelled words in the space provided. Sign your work and give it to your instructor. You are now ready for the next lesson.

PRACTICE

LESSON

17

Terminology Presentation

Listen to the Lab Tape provided by your instructor, and you will hear the words presented in this lesson. Read the words as they are said, noticing spelling and pronunciation. The recording will tell you when the presentation for this lesson is completed and will give you any further instructions. Do not go on to the next recorded lesson until you have completed Lesson 17 and feel that you know the words and word parts that have been presented.

• • • ▸ *Start Audio*

oophor(o) a word part denoting the ovaries

WORD	WORD PART	DEFINITION	ANSWER
1. oophorocystosis (o-of'o-ro-sis-to'sis)	cyst -osis	sac, cyst condition, process, increase, disease	1. ________
2. oophoroma (o-of'o-ro'mah)	-oma	tumor	2. ________
3. oophoritis (o'of-o-ri'tis)	-itis	inflammation	3. ________
4. oophorectomy (o'of-o-rek'to-me)	-ectomy	excision, removal	4. ________
5. oophorostomy (o-of'o-ros'to-me)	-ostomy	opening	5. ________
6. oophoroplasty (o-of'o-ro-plas'te)	-plasty	plastic surgery	6. ________
7. oophorrhagia (o-of'o-ra'je-ah)	-rrhagia	excessive flow, bleeding	7. ________

salping(o) a word element denoting the uterine (fallopian) tube or auditory (eustachian) tube

WORD	WORD PART	DEFINITION	ANSWER
8. salpingitis (sal'pin-ji'tis)	-itis	inflammation	8. ________

9. salpingocele (sal-ping'go-sel)	-cele	tumor, swelling, hernia	9. ________
10. salpingocyesis (sal-ping'go-si-e'sis)	-cyesis	pregnancy	10. ________
11. salpingo-oophorectomy (sal-ping'go-o'of-o-rek'to-me)	oophor(o)	ovaries	11. ________
	-ectomy	excision, removal	
12. salpingotomy (sal-ping-got'o-me)	-otomy	incision, cutting into	12. ________
13. salpingorrhagia (sal-ping'go-ra'je-ah)	-rrhagia	excessive flow, bleeding	13. ________
14. salpingography (sal'ping-gog'rah-fe)	-graphy	recording	14. ________
15. salpingoscopy (sal'ping-gos'ko-pe)	-scopy	examine	15. ________
16. salpingorrhaphy (sal'ping-gor'ah-fe)	-rrhaphy	suture, surgical repair	16. ________
17. salpingemphraxis (sal'pin-jem-frak'sis)	-emphraxis	stoppage	17. ________

■ • • • *Stop Audio at Tone*

Study the 17 words and word parts for this lesson. Practice each word several times, checking your spelling and repeating the meaning to yourself. Listen to the recording and pronounce the words as many times as necessary. When you feel that you know the words and word parts well, you are ready to go on to the next step.

Use a sheet of paper to cover all columns except the Answer Column on the previous page. The words you have learned will be presented again on the recording. As each word is pronounced, write it in the space provided in the Answer Column.

• • • ▸ *Start Audio*

After stopping the tape player, check the words you have written against the words in the left-hand column. If any words are misspelled, practice writing them correctly. When you feel that you know and understand the words and word parts, go on to the Terminology Practice.

PRACTICE

____

____

____

Name ______________________ Date ______________ Errors ________

LESSON 17: TERMINOLOGY PRACTICE

Without looking at your previous work, write the word that is described by each definition.

oophor(o) and *salping(o)*

DEFINITION	TERM
1. Visual examination of the uterine tube	________
2. Inflammation of the uterine tube (canal) or auditory tube (canal)	________
3. Excision or surgical removal of an ovary	________
4. Hernial protrusion of a uterine tube	________
5. Tumor of the ovary	________
6. The formation of an ovarian cyst	________
7. Surgical incision into the uterine tube	________
8. Hemorrhage or bleeding from an ovary	________
9. Plastic surgery on the ovary	________
10. The making of an opening into an ovarian cyst to provide drainage	________
11. Excision of the ovary and the uterine tube	________
12. Hemorrhage from a fallopian tube	________
13. Inflammation of an ovary	________
14. Tubal pregnancy	________
15. Roentgenogram or x-ray picture of the uterine tube or tubes	________
16. Obstruction of a uterine or eustachian tube	________
17. Suture or surgical repair of the uterine tube	________

Check your answers against the word and definition lists on the first page of this lesson. If you have any errors, count them and write the number in the blank at the top of the page. Practice any missed or misspelled words in the space provided. Sign your work and give it to your instructor. You are now ready for the next lesson.

PRACTICE

LESSON

18 Terminology Presentation

Listen to the Lab Tape provided by your instructor, and you will hear the words presented in this lesson. Read the words as they are said, noticing spelling and pronunciation. The recording will tell you when the presentation for this lesson is completed and will give you any further instructions. Do not go on to the next recorded lesson until you have completed Lesson 18 and feel that you know the words and word parts that have been presented.

• • • ▶ *Start Audio*

metr(o), metr(a) a combining form denoting the uterus

WORD	WORD PART	DEFINITION	ANSWER
1. metritis (me-tri′tis)	-itis	inflammation	1. ________
2. metrocolpocele (me′tro-kol′po-sel)	colp(o) -cele	vagina tumor, swelling, hernia	2. ________
3. metrorrhea (me′tro-re′ah)	-rrhea	flow	3. ________
4. metropathy (me-trop′ah-the)	-pathy	disease	4. ________
5. metrostenosis (me′tro-ste-no′sis)	-stenosis	narrowing	5. ________
6. metroptosis (me′tro-to′sis)	-ptosis	falling	6. ________
7. metrorrhagia (me′tro-ra′je-ah)	-rrhagia	excessive flow, bleeding	7. ________

gyn(o), gynec(o) a word element denoting women or the female sex

WORD	WORD PART	DEFINITION	ANSWER
8. gynecology (gi′ne-kol′o-je)	-logy	study of, science of	8. ________

9. gynandromorphous (ji-nan'dro-mor'fus)	andro morph(ous)	man, male shape, form	9. ______
10. gynecomastia (jin'e-ko-mas'te-ah)	mast(o)	breast, mammary gland	10. ______
11. gynecologist (gi'ne-kol'o-jist)	-logist	specialist	11. ______
12. gynopathy (jin-op'ah-the)	-pathy	disease	12. ______
13. gynephobia (jin'e-fo'be-ah)	-phobia	fear	13. ______
14. gynoplasty (ji'no-plas'te)	-plasty	plastic surgery	14. ______

■ • • • *Stop Audio at Tone*

Study the 14 words and word parts for this lesson. Practice each word several times, checking your spelling and repeating the meaning to yourself. Listen to the recording and pronounce the words as many times as necessary. When you feel that you know the words and word parts well, you are ready to go on to the next step.

Use a sheet of paper to cover all columns except the Answer Column on the previous page. The words you have learned will be presented again on the recording. As each word is pronounced, write it in the space provided in the Answer Column.

• • • ▸ *Start Audio*

After stopping the tape player, check the words you have written against the words in the left-hand column. If any words are misspelled, practice writing them correctly. When you feel that you know and understand the words and word parts, go on to the Terminology Practice.

PRACTICE

____

____

____

____

____

____

____

____

Name ______________________ Date ______________ Errors ________

LESSON 18: TERMINOLOGY PRACTICE

Without looking at your previous work, write the word that is described by each definition.

metr(o), metr(a) and ***gyn(o), gynec(o)***

DEFINITION	TERM
1. A narrowing of the uterine cavity	______________
2. Plastic surgery on the female organs	______________
3. Inflammation of the uterus	______________
4. Excessive development of the male mammary glands or breasts	______________
5. Uterine bleeding	______________
6. Specialist in treating female disorders	______________
7. Hernial protrusion of the uterus into the vagina	______________
8. A discharge of mucus or pus from the uterus	______________
9. Any disease of women	______________
10. Any uterine disease	______________
11. A morbid fear of women	______________
12. The branch of medicine treating diseases of women	______________
13. Having both male and female qualities	______________
14. Prolapse of the uterus	______________

Check your answers against the word and definition lists on the first page of this lesson. If you have any errors, count them and write the number in the blank at the top of the page. Practice any missed or misspelled words on the next page. Sign your work and give it to your instructor. You are now ready for the next lesson.

PRACTICE

LESSON

19

Terminology Presentation

Listen to the Lab Tape provided by your instructor, and you will hear the words presented in this lesson. Read the words as they are said, noticing spelling and pronunciation. The recording will tell you when the presentation for this lesson is completed and will give you any further instructions. Do not go on to the next recorded lesson until you have completed Lesson 19 and feel that you know the words and word parts that have been presented.

• • • ▸ *Start Audio*

nephr(o) a combining form denoting relationship to the kidney

WORD	WORD PART	DEFINITION	ANSWER
1. nephritis (ne-fri′tis)	-itis	inflammation	1. ________
2. pyelonephritis (pi′e-lo-ne-fri′tis)	pyel(o) -itis	pelvis of the kidney inflammation	2. ________
3. nephrohydrosis (nef′ro-hi-dro′sis)	hydr(o) -osis	water, fluid condition, process, increase, disease	3. ________
4. nephrolithiasis (nef′ro-li-thi′ah-sis)	-lithiasis	stone	4. ________
5. nephrapostasis (nef′rah-pos′tah-sis)	-apostasis	suppuration, pus	5. ________
6. nephropathy (ne-frop′ah-the)	-pathy	disease	6. ________
7. nephroptosis (nef′rop-to′sis)	-ptosis	falling	7. ________
8. nephrology (ne-frol′o-je)	-(o)logy	study of, science of	8. ________

hyster(o) a combining form denoting the uterus

WORD	WORD PART	DEFINITION	ANSWER
9. hysterectomy (his′te-rek′to-me)	-ectomy	excision, removal	9. ________

10. hysterocleisis (his′ter-o-kli′sis)	-cleisis	closure	**10.** ________
11. hysteralgia (his′te-ral′je-ah)	-algia	pain	**11.** ________
12. hysterospasm (his′ter-o-spazm′)	-spasm	contraction	**12.** ________
13. hysterotracheloplasty (his′ter-o-tra′kel-o-plas′te)	trachel(o) -plasty	cervix, neck plastic surgery	**13.** ________
14. hysterostomatomy (his′ter-o-sto-mat′o-me)	stom(a) -tomy	mouth, opening incision, cutting into	**14.** ________
15. hysteropexy (his′ter-o-pek-se)	-pexy	fix, fasten	**15.** ________
16. hysterocolposcope (his′ter-o-kol′po-skop)	colp(o) -scope	vagina viewing instrument	**16.** ________

■ • • • *Stop Audio at Tone*

Study the 16 words and word parts for this lesson. Practice each word several times, checking your spelling and repeating the meaning to yourself. Listen to the recording and pronounce the words as many times as necessary. When you feel that you know the words and word parts well, you are ready to go on to the next step.

Use a sheet of paper to cover all columns except the Answer Column on the previous page. The words you have learned will be presented again on the recording. As each word is pronounced, write it in the space provided in the Answer Column.

• • • ▶ *Start Audio*

After stopping the tape player, check the words you have written against the words in the left-hand column. If any words are misspelled, practice writing them correctly. When you feel that you know and understand the words and word parts, go on to the Terminology Practice.

PRACTICE

Name ______________________ Date ______________ Errors ________

LESSON 19: TERMINOLOGY PRACTICE

Without looking at your previous work, write the word that is described by each definition.

nephr(o) and *hyster(o)*

DEFINITION	TERM
1. Surgical closure of the os uteri	______________
2. Removal or excision of the uterus	______________
3. Downward displacement of the kidney	______________
4. Inflammation of the kidney and its pelvis	______________
5. Any kidney disease	______________
6. An instrument for inspection of the uterine cavity and vagina	______________
7. Pain in the uterus	______________
8. A uterine spasm	______________
9. Abscess of the kidney with suppuration	______________
10. Inflammation of the kidney	______________
11. Surgical fixation or fastening of the uterus	______________
12. Plastic repair of the cervix uteri	______________
13. Kidney stones	______________
14. Study of the kidney and its diseases	______________
15. An accumulation of water or fluid in the kidneys	______________
16. Incision into the mouth of the uterus	______________

Check your answers against the word and definition lists on the first page of this lesson. If you have any errors, count them and write the number in the blank at the top of the page. Practice any missed or misspelled words in the space provided. Sign your work and give it to your instructor. You are now ready for the next lesson.

PRACTICE

Name ________________________ Date ________________ Errors ________

LESSON 20 | TERMINOLOGY REVIEW FOR TEST 4

This is a review of the word parts you have learned in the preceding four lessons. Some of the medical terms listed below may be new, but they are made up of word parts that you have already learned.

Unlike the review for Test 3, the words are not written out for you. As each word is pronounced on the Lab Tape, write it in the appropriate numbered blank on the left.

• • • ▶ *Start Audio*

WORD	WORD PART	MEANING OF WORD PART
1. ____________	____________	____________
	____________	____________
	____________	____________
2. ____________	____________	____________
	____________	____________
3. ____________	____________	____________
	____________	____________
	____________	____________
4. ____________	____________	____________
	____________	____________
	____________	____________
5. ____________	____________	____________
	____________	____________
	____________	____________
6. ____________	____________	____________
	____________	____________
	____________	____________
7. ____________	____________	____________
	____________	____________
	____________	____________
8. ____________	____________	____________
	____________	____________
	____________	____________

9. ______________________ ______________ ________________________________
______________ ________________________________
______________ ________________________________

10. ______________________ ______________ ________________________________
______________ ________________________________
______________ ________________________________

11. ______________________ ______________ ________________________________
______________ ________________________________
______________ ________________________________

12. ______________________ ______________ ________________________________
______________ ________________________________
______________ ________________________________

13. ______________________ ______________ ________________________________
______________ ________________________________
______________ ________________________________

14. ______________________ ______________ ________________________________
______________ ________________________________
______________ ________________________________

15. ______________________ ______________ ________________________________
______________ ________________________________
______________ ________________________________

■ • • • *Stop Audio at Tone*

After all 15 words have been written, write the word parts for each one and fill in the meanings of the parts. Use the Glossary or a dictionary to check your spellings and definitions. Practice the words on a separate sheet of paper, paying particular attention to any you missed or misspelled.

When you feel you know the words and word parts well, sign your work, indicate the number of errors, and turn your work in to your instructor.

You are now ready for the Extra Credit Review (if your instructor assigns it) or Test 4.

Name ______________________ Date ______________ Errors ________

LESSON 20 **EXTRA CREDIT REVIEW**

This Extra Credit Review should be done at the discretion of your instructor. If you are instructed to complete this portion of the Review, turn it in to your instructor when you are finished.

PART A

Write the definition for the following 20 terms to the right of the given term.

TERM	DEFINITION
1. pyelitis	______________________
2. oophorostomy	______________________
3. nocturia	______________________
4. salpingemphraxis	______________________
5. metrorrhea	______________________
6. pyelocystitis	______________________
7. gynephobia	______________________
8. bacteriuria	______________________
9. oophoritis	______________________
10. salpingography	______________________
11. nephrolithiasis	______________________
12. polyuria	______________________
13. gynandromorphous	______________________
14. salpingorrhagia	______________________
15. hysterocleisis	______________________
16. metrostenosis	______________________
17. pyelolithotomy	______________________
18. nephroptosis	______________________

19. hysteralgia ______________________________

20. gynecology ______________________________

PART B

Match the following definitions with the terms given. Place the correct letter of the definition to the left of the term.

TERM

______ 21. albuminuria

______ 22. metrocolpocele

______ 23. nephropathy

______ 24. salpingoscopy

______ 25. pyelophlebitis

______ 26. gynecomastia

______ 27. hysterotracheloplasty

______ 28. metrostenosis

______ 29. nephrohydrosis

______ 30. oophorocystosis

DEFINITION

a. the formation of an ovarian cyst
b. inflammation of the veins of the renal pelvis and bladder
c. presence of serum albumin in the urine
d. hernial protrusion of the uterus into the vagina
e. any kidney disease
f. visual examination of the uterine tube
g. plastic repair of the cervix uteri
h. a narrowing of the uterine cavity
i. excessive development of the male mammary glands or breasts
j. an accumulation of water or fluid in the kidney

You may now go on to Test 4.

SECTION

5 Nervous System

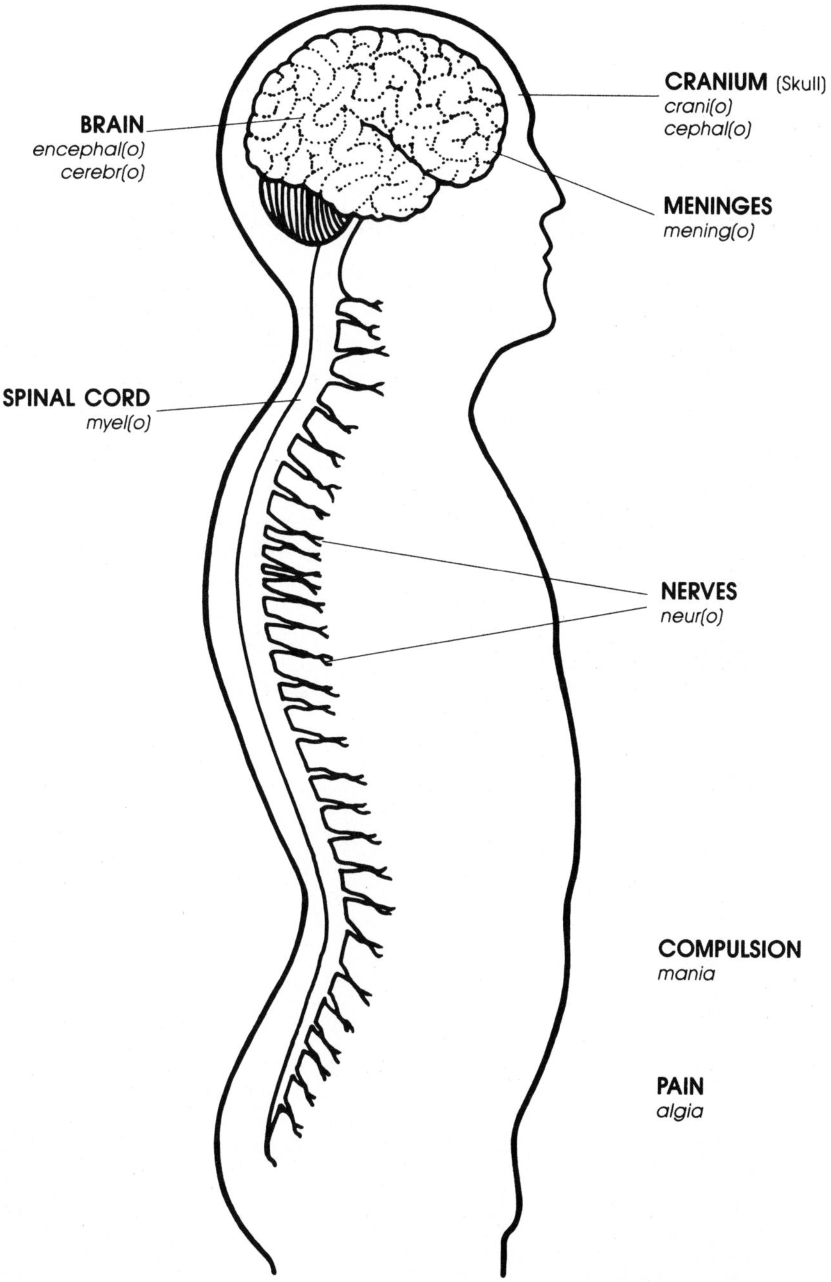

NERVOUS SYSTEM

Orientation

The nervous system consists of two main parts, the central nervous system and the peripheral nervous system. The central nervous system (CNS) is composed of the brain and spinal cord. It is responsible for coordinating the actions of the voluntary muscles (body movement) and the conscious thought processes (thinking, feeling, and emotions). The brain contains 12 billion cells and is a very complicated communications center for the body. It is divided into three parts—the brain stem, cerebrum, and cerebellum. The brain stem is connected to the lower part of the brain. Impulses of all kinds travel up and down this column, sending messages to and from the brain.

The peripheral nervous system is made up of 31 pairs of spinal nerves, which are bundles of nerve cells or neurons. These nerves are the message-relaying mechanism for the brain. Afferent nerves note changes within the body and in the outside environment, and they signal these changes to the brain by means of electrical impulses. The brain interprets the nerve impulses and in turn sends "action" messages to all parts of the body via efferent nerves.

Some of the body's nerves are involved in the autonomic nervous system, which controls the organs, glands, and certain muscles automatically. The autonomic nervous system is further divided into sympathetic and parasympathetic nerves. The sympathetic nerves prepare the body for stress and action in times of emergency by slowing digestion and increasing the heart rate, respiration, and blood pressure. The parasympathetic nerves restore the body's systems to "normal" after the emergency is over by lowering blood pressure, slowing breathing, decreasing the heart rate, and stimulating digestion.

All parts of the nervous system are interdependent and work with each other. The brain is the most complex computer known.

LESSON 21

Terminology Presentation

Listen to the Lab Tape provided by your instructor, and you will hear the words presented in this lesson. Read the words as they are said, noticing spelling and pronunciation. The recording will tell you when the presentation for this lesson is completed and will give you any further instructions. Do not go on to the next recorded lesson until you have completed Lesson 21 and feel that you know the words and word parts that have been presented.

• • • ▸ *Start Audio*

myel, myel(o) a word part denoting spinal cord or bone marrow

WORD	WORD PART	DEFINITION	ANSWER
1. myelauxe (mi′el-awks′e)	-auxe	increase	1. ______
2. myelocele (mi′e-lo-sel)	-cele	tumor, swelling, hernia	2. ______
3. poliomyelitis (po′le-o-mi′e-li′tis)	polio	gray	3. ______
4. myelocyte (mi′e-lo-sit)	-cyte	cell	4. ______
5. myelomalacia (mi′e-lo-mah-la′she-ah)	-malacia	softening	5. ______
6. myeloplegia (mi′e-lo-ple′je-ah)	-plegia	paralysis	6. ______
7. myelophthisis (mi′e-lof′thi-sis)	-phthisis	wasting	7. ______
8. myelogenous (mi′e-loj′e-nus)	-genous	to produce	8. ______

crani(o) a combining form denoting the skull or cranium

WORD	WORD PART	DEFINITION	ANSWER
9. craniectomy (kra′ne-ek′to-me)	-ectomy	excision, removal	9. ______

10. craniocele (kra′ne-o-sel′)	-cele	tumor, swelling, hernia	10. ______
11. craniomalacia (kra′ne-o-mah-la′she-ah)	-malacia	softening	11. ______
12. craniotomy kra′ne-ot′o-me)	-(o)tomy	incision, cutting into	12. ______
13. craniorachischisis (kra′ne-o-rah-kis′ki-sis)	rach(i) -schisis	spine splitting	13. ______
14. cranioplasty (kra′ne-o-plas′te)	-plasty	plastic surgery	14. ______
15. craniospinal (kra′ne-o-spi′nal)	-spin(al)	spine	15. ______

■ • • • *Stop Audio at Tone*

Study the 15 words and word parts for this lesson. Practice each word several times, checking your spelling and repeating the meaning to yourself. Listen to the recording and pronounce the words as many times as necessary. When you feel that you know the words and word parts well, you are ready to go on to the next step.

Use a sheet of paper to cover all columns except the Answer Column on the previous page. The words you have learned will be presented again on the recording. As each word is pronounced, write it in the space provided in the Answer Column.

• • • ▶ *Start Audio*

After stopping the tape player, check the words you have written against the words in the left-hand column. If any words are misspelled, practice writing them correctly. When you feel that you know and understand the words and word parts, go on to the Terminology Practice.

PRACTICE

______

______

______

______

______

______

______

______

Name ______________________ Date ______________ Errors ________

LESSON 21: TERMINOLOGY PRACTICE

Without looking at your previous work, write the word that is described by each definition.

myel(o) and *crani(o)*

DEFINITION	TERM
1. Wasting of the spinal cord	______________
2. Inflammation of the gray matter of the spinal cord	______________
3. An operation on or incision into the skull	______________
4. Softening of the skull	______________
5. A protrusion of part of the cranial contents through a defect in the skull	______________
6. Produced in the bone marrow	______________
7. Morbid softening of the spinal cord	______________
8. Removal or excision of a part of the skull	______________
9. Morbid increase in the size of the spinal cord	______________
10. Swelling or hernial protrusion of the spinal cord	______________
11. Plastic surgery on the cranium	______________
12. A marrow cell	______________
13. Pertaining to the skull and spine	______________
14. Congenital fissure of the skull and spinal column	______________
15. Paralysis of the spinal cord or spinal paralysis	______________

Check your answers against the word and definition lists on the first page of this lesson. If you have any errors, count them and write the number in the blank at the top of the page. Practice any missed or misspelled words on the next page. Sign your work and give it to your instructor. You are now ready for the next lesson.

PRACTICE

LESSON 22

Terminology Presentation

Listen to the Lab Tape provided by your instructor, and you will hear the words presented in this lesson. Read the words as they are said, noticing spelling and pronunciation. The recording will tell you when the presentation for this lesson is completed and will give you any further instructions. Do not go on to the next recorded lesson until you have completed Lesson 22 and feel that you know the words and word parts that have been presented.

• • • ▶ *Start Audio*

encephal(o) a combining form denoting the brain (en: inside or within, combined with cephal: head)

WORD	WORD PART	DEFINITION	ANSWER
1. encephalodysplasia (en-sef'ah-lo-dis-pla'se-ah)	dys -plasia	abnormal, painful formation	1. ________
2. encephalitis (en'sef-ah-li'tis)	-itis	inflammation	2. ________
3. encephalogram (en-sef'ah-lo-gram')	-gram	something recorded	3. ________
4. encephalothlipsis (en-sef'a-lo-thlip'sis)	-thlipsis	pressure	4. ________
5. encephalopathic (en-sef'ah-lo-path'ik)	path(o) -ic	disease pertaining to	5. ________
6. encephaloma (en'sef-ah-lo'mah)	-oma	tumor	6. ________
7. encephalomalacia (en-sef'ah-lo-mah-la'she-ah)	-malacia	softening	7. ________

psych(o), psych a word part denoting the mind or the mental faculties

WORD	WORD PART	DEFINITION	ANSWER
8. psychataxia (si'kah-tak'se-ah)	-ataxia	confusion	8. ________

9. psychogenic (si'ko-jen'ik)	-genic	produce	9. ________
10. psychoneurosis (si'ko-nu-ro'sis)	neur(o) -osis	nerves condition, process, increase, disease	10. ________
11. psychasthenia (si'kas-the'ne-ah)	a- -sthenia	without, lack of strength	11. ________
12. psychology (si'kol'o-je)	-ology	study of, science of	12. ________
13. psychosomatic (si'ko-so-mat'ik)	somat(o) -ic	body pertaining to	13. ________
14. psychotherapy (si-ko-ther'ah-pe)	-therapy	treatment	14. ________
15. psychophylaxis (si'ko-fi-lak'sis)	-phylaxis	protection	15. ________

■ • • • *Stop Audio at Tone*

Study the 15 words and word parts for this lesson. Practice each word several times, checking your spelling and repeating the meaning to yourself. Listen to the recording and pronounce the words as many times as necessary. When you feel that you know the words and word parts well, you are ready to go on to the next step.

Use a sheet of paper to cover all columns except the Answer Column on the previous page. The words you have learned will be presented again on the recording. As each word is pronounced, write it in the space provided in the Answer Column.

• • • ▶ *Start Audio*

After stopping the tape player, check the words you have written against the words in the left-hand column. If any words are misspelled, practice writing them correctly. When you feel that you know and understand the words and word parts, go on to the Terminology Practice.

PRACTICE

____

____

____

____

____

Name ______________________ Date ______________ Errors ________

LESSON 22: TERMINOLOGY PRACTICE

Without looking at your previous work, write the word that is described by each definition.

encephal(o) and *psych(o), psych*

DEFINITION	TERM
1. X-ray picture of the brain	______________
2. Preventing mental illness	______________
3. Any congenital abnormality of the brain	______________
4. Inflammation of the brain	______________
5. Treatment of emotional, behavioral, and mental disorders	______________
6. The branch of medicine that studies the mind	______________
7. Morbid softening of the brain tissue	______________
8. Compression of the brain	______________
9. A term to denote a functional personality disorder literally translated as mental weakness	______________
10. Originating or developing in the mind	______________
11. Mental confusion, inability to fix the attention	______________
12. A brain tumor	______________
13. A mental or behavioral disorder which presents symptoms of functional nervous disease	______________
14. Pertaining to the mind-body relationship	______________
15. Pertaining to a brain disease	______________

Check your answers against the word and definition lists on the first page of this lesson. If you have any errors, count them and write the number in the blank at the top of the page. Practice any missed or misspelled words on the next page. Sign your work and give it to your instructor. You are now ready for the next lesson.

PRACTICE

LESSON

23 Terminology Presentation

Listen to the Lab Tape provided by your instructor, and you will hear the words presented in this lesson. Read the words as they are said, noticing spelling and pronunciation. The recording will tell you when the presentation for this lesson is completed and will give you any further instructions. Do not go on to the next recorded lesson until you have completed Lesson 23 and feel that you know the words and word parts that have been presented.

••• ▶ *Start Audio*

algia, algesia a word element (suffix, usually) denoting pain or ache

WORD	WORD PART	DEFINITION	ANSWER
1. dermalgia (der-mal′je-ah)	derm(o)	skin	1. ____________
2. odontalgia (o-don-tal′je-ah)	odont(o)	tooth	2. ____________
3. arthralgia (ar-thral′je-ah)	arthr(o)	joint	3. ____________
4. otalgia (o-tal′je-ah)	ot(o)	ear	4. ____________
5. hyperalgesia (hi′per-al-je′ze-ah)	hyper-	above, over, abundant	5. ____________
6. analgesic (an′al-je′zik)	an -ic	without, lack of pertaining to	6. ____________
7. gastralgia (gas-tral′je-ah)	gastr(o)	stomach	7. ____________
8. myalgia (mi-al′je-ah)	my(o)	muscle	8. ____________
9. kinesalgia (kin′e-sal′je-ah)	kines	motion	9. ____________
10. costalgia (kos-tal′je-ah)	cost(o)	rib	10. ____________

mania, manic a word ending (suffix) denoting an abnormal love for or compulsion

WORD	WORD PART	DEFINITION	ANSWER
11. kleptomania (klep′to-ma′ne-ah)	klept(o)	to steal	11. __________
12. pyromania (pi′ro-ma′ne-ah)	pyr(o)	heat, fire	12. __________
13. megalomania (meg′ah-lo-ma′ne-ah)	megal(o)	large, great	13. __________
14. erotomania (e-rot′o-ma′ne-ah)	erot(o)	love	14. __________
15. oniomania (o′ne-o-ma′ne-ah)	oni(o)	for sale	15. __________

■ • • • *Stop Audio at Tone*

Study the 15 words and word parts for this lesson. Practice each word several times, checking your spelling and repeating the meaning to yourself. Listen to the recording and pronounce the words as many times as necessary. When you feel that you know the words and word parts well, you are ready to go on to the next step.

Use a sheet of paper to cover all columns except the Answer Column on the previous page. The words you have learned will be presented again on the recording. As each word is pronounced, write it in the space provided in the Answer Column.

• • • ▶ *Start Audio*

After stopping the tape player, check the words you have written against the words in the left-hand column. If any words are misspelled, practice writing them correctly. When you feel that you know and understand the words and word parts, go on to the Terminology Practice.

PRACTICE

____

____

____

____

____

____

Name ______________________ Date ________________ Errors ________

LESSON 23: TERMINOLOGY PRACTICE

Without looking at your previous work, write the word that is described by each definition.

algia, algesia or *mania, manic*

DEFINITION	TERM
1. Pain in the stomach, stomachache	________________
2. Rib pain	________________
3. Delusions of grandeur, unreasonable conviction of one's own greatness	________________
4. Pain on motion or movement	________________
5. A morbid compulsion to set fires	________________
6. Increased sensation to pain	________________
7. Earache, pain in the ear	________________
8. A morbid desire to buy beyond one's realistic needs (shop till you drop)	________________
9. Skin pain	________________
10. A compulsion to steal	________________
11. Muscle pain	________________
12. Toothache	________________
13. Excessive or morbid inclination to erotic thoughts or behavior	________________
14. Painful joints	________________
15. Pertaining to the giving of a medicine to relieve or remove pain	________________

Check your answers against the word and definition lists on the first page of this lesson. If you have any errors, count them and write the number in the blank at the top of the page. Practice any missed or misspelled words on the next page. Sign your work and give it to your instructor. You are now ready for the next lesson.

PRACTICE

LESSON 24

Terminology Presentation

Listen to the Lab Tape provided by your instructor, and you will hear the words presented in this lesson. Read the words as they are said, noticing spelling and pronunciation. The recording will tell you when the presentation for this lesson is completed and will give you any further instructions. Do not go on to the next recorded lesson until you have completed Lesson 24 and feel that you know the words and word parts that have been presented.

• • • ▸ *Start Audio*

neur(o) a combining form denoting the nerves or nervous system

WORD	WORD PART	DEFINITION	ANSWER
1. neurobiology (nu′ro-bi-ol′o-je)	bi(o) -ology	life study of, science of	1. ________
2. neuralgia (nu-ral′je-ah)	-algia	pain	2. ________
3. neuritis (nu-ri′tis)	-itis	inflammation	3. ________
4. neuroma (nu-ro′mah)	-oma	tumor	4. ________
5. neuragmia (nu-rag′me-ah)	-agmia	break or tear	5. ________
6. neuropathy (nu-rop′ah-the)	-pathy	disease	6. ________
7. neurosis (nu-ro′sis)	-osis	condition, process, increase, disease	7. ________
8. neurooncology (nu′ro-on-kol′o-je)	onc(o) -ology	tumor study of, science of	8. ________

cephal(o) a combining form indicating the cranium (head) or the head of a body part

WORD	WORD PART	DEFINITION	ANSWER
9. cephaledema (sef′al-e-de′mah)	-edema	swelling	9. ________

10. cephalocele (se-fal′o-sel)	-cele	tumor, swelling, hernia	**10.** ________
11. cephaloplegia (sef′ah-lo-ple′je-ah)	-plegia	paralysis	**11.** ________
12. cephalometer (sef′ah-lom′e-ter)	-meter	measure	**12.** ________
13. cephalocentesis (sef′ah-lo-sen-te′sis)	-centesis	surgical puncture	**13.** ________
14. cephalic (se-fal′ik)	-ic	pertaining to	**14.** ________
15. cephalocaudal (sef′ah-lo-kaw′dal)	caud(o) -al	tail pertaining to	**15.** ________

■ • • • *Stop Audio at Tone*

Study the 15 words and word parts for this lesson. Practice each word several times, checking your spelling and repeating the meaning to yourself. Listen to the recording and pronounce the words as many times as necessary. When you feel that you know the words and word parts well, you are ready to go on to the next step.

Use a sheet of paper to cover all columns except the Answer Column on the previous page. The words you have learned will be presented again on the recording. As each word is pronounced, write it in the space provided in the Answer Column.

• • • ▸ *Start Audio*

After stopping the tape player, check the words you have written against the words in the left-hand column. If any words are misspelled, practice writing them correctly. When you feel that you know and understand the words and word parts, go on to the Terminology Practice.

PRACTICE

____

____

____

____

____

____

____

____

Name ______________________ Date ______________ Errors ________

LESSON 24: TERMINOLOGY PRACTICE

Without looking at your previous work, write the word that is described by each definition.

neur(o) and *cephal(o)*

DEFINITION	TERM
1. The study of tumors of the nervous system	________
2. Tumor composed of nerve cells	________
3. Hernial protrusion of part of the cranial contents	________
4. The tearing of a nerve	________
5. Paralysis of the head muscles	________
6. The biology of the nervous system	________
7. Surgical puncture of the skull or head to draw off fluid	________
8. Instrument to measure the head	________
9. Nerve pain	________
10. Pertaining to the long axis of the body (head to tail)	________
11. Inflammation of a nerve	________
12. Any disease of the nerves	________
13. Swelling or edema of the head	________
14. An emotional (nervous) disorder characterized by anxiety	________
15. Pertaining to the head	________

Check your answers against the word and definition lists on the first page of this lesson. If you have any errors, count them and write the number in the blank at the top of the page. Practice any missed or misspelled words on the next page. Sign your work and give it to your instructor. You are now ready for the next lesson.

PRACTICE

Name ______________________ Date ______________ Errors ________

LESSON 25 — TERMINOLOGY REVIEW FOR TEST 5

This is a review of the word parts you have learned in the preceding four lessons. Some of the medical terms listed below may be new, but they are made up of word parts that you have already learned. Read the words below as they are pronounced on the Lab Tape. As you listen, notice the familiar word parts which make them up.

• • • ▸ ***Start Audio***

WORD	WORD PART	MEANING OF WORD PART
1. craniomalacia	crani(o)	______
(kra′ne-o-mah-la′she-ah)	-malacia	______
craniomalacia	______	
2. neuroma	neur(o)	______
(nu-ro′mah)	-oma	______
neuroma	______	
3. cephalocaudal	cephal(o)	______
(sef′ah-lo-kaw′dal)	caud(o)	______
	-al	______
cephalocaudal	______	
4. myelogenous	myel(o)	______
(mi′e-loj′e-nus)	-genous	______
myelogenous	______	
5. neuralgia	neur(o)	______
(nu-ral′je-ah)	-algia	______
neuralgia	______	
6. cephalocele	cephal(o)	______
(se-fal′o-sel)	-cele	______
cephalocele	______	
7. odontalgia	odont(o)	______
(o-don-tal′je-ah)	-algia	______
odontalgia	______	
8. psychology	psych(o)	______
(si′kol′o-je)	-ology	______
psychology	______	

9. cephaloplegia (sef′ah-lo-ple′je-ah)
cephal(o) ______________________
-plegia ______________________
cephaloplegia ______________________

10. hyperalgesia (hi′per-al-je′ze-ah)
hyper- ______________________
-algesia ______________________
hyperalgesia ______________________

11. myelauxe (mi′el-awks′e)
myel(o) ______________________
-auxe ______________________
myelauxe ______________________

12. craniorachischisis (kra′ne-o-rah-kis′ki-sis)
crani(o) ______________________
rachi ______________________
-schisis ______________________
craniorachischisis ______________________

13. oniomania (o′ne-o-ma′ne-ah)
oni(o) ______________________
-mania ______________________
oniomania ______________________

14. encephalodysplasia (en-sef′ah-lo-dis-pla′se-ah)
encephal(o) ______________________
dys ______________________
-plasia ______________________
encephalodysplasia ______________________

15. neurooncology (nu′ro-on-kol′o-je)
neur(o) ______________________
onc(o) ______________________
-ology ______________________
neurooncology ______________________

■ • • • *Stop Audio at Tone*

On the lines provided, fill in the meanings of as many of the word parts as you can from memory. Then, use the previous lessons or a medical dictionary to look up any definitions you could not remember. Fill them in. On a separate piece of paper, practice writing the word parts and their meanings. Pay special attention to any which you had trouble remembering. Be sure to check your spelling.

When you have defined and reviewed all the word parts, write a definition for each whole word on the line provided. Check your definitions in the Glossary or a medical dictionary and make any needed corrections. Practice the words on a separate sheet of paper until you are sure that you know them. Then go on to the Extra Credit Review (if your instructor assigns it) or Test 5.

Name ______________________ Date ______________ Errors ________

LESSON 25 — EXTRA CREDIT REVIEW

This Extra Credit Review should be done at the discretion of your instructor. If you are instructed to complete this portion of the Review, turn your paper in to your instructor when you are finished.

PART A

Each phrase below defines one of the words you have just studied. Without looking at your previous work, fill in the word that matches each definition.

DEFINITION	TERM
1. The study of tumors of the nervous system	________________
2. Produced in the bone marrow	________________
3. Increased sensation to pain	________________
4. Any congenital abnormality of the brain	________________
5. Hernial protrusion of part of the cranial contents	________________
6. Morbid softening of the cranium	________________
7. Congenital fissure of the skull and spinal column	________________
8. Tumor of nerve cells	________________
9. Toothache	________________
10. Pertaining to the long axis of the body	________________
11. Morbid increase in the size of the spinal cord	________________
12. The branch of medicine treating the mind	________________
13. Nerve pain	________________
14. A morbid desire to buy beyond one's realistic needs	________________
15. Paralysis of the head muscles	________________

PART B

Match the following terms with the definitions given. Place the correct letter of the term to the left of the definition.

DEFINITION	TERM
______ **16.** A marrow cell	a. psychataxia
	b. encephalitis
______ **17.** Pertaining to the skull and spine	c. costalgia
	d. myelophthisis
______ **18.** Mental confusion, inability to fix the attention	e. myelocyte
	f. cephaledema
______ **19.** Stomach pain	g. craniospinal
	h. gastralgia
______ **20.** A compulsion to steal	i. kleptomania
	j. neuragmia
______ **21.** Inflammation of the brain	
______ **22.** Wasting of the spinal cord	
______ **23.** The tearing of a nerve	
______ **24.** Rib pain	
______ **25.** Swelling or edema of the head	

You may now go on to Test 5.

SECTION

6 Respiratory System

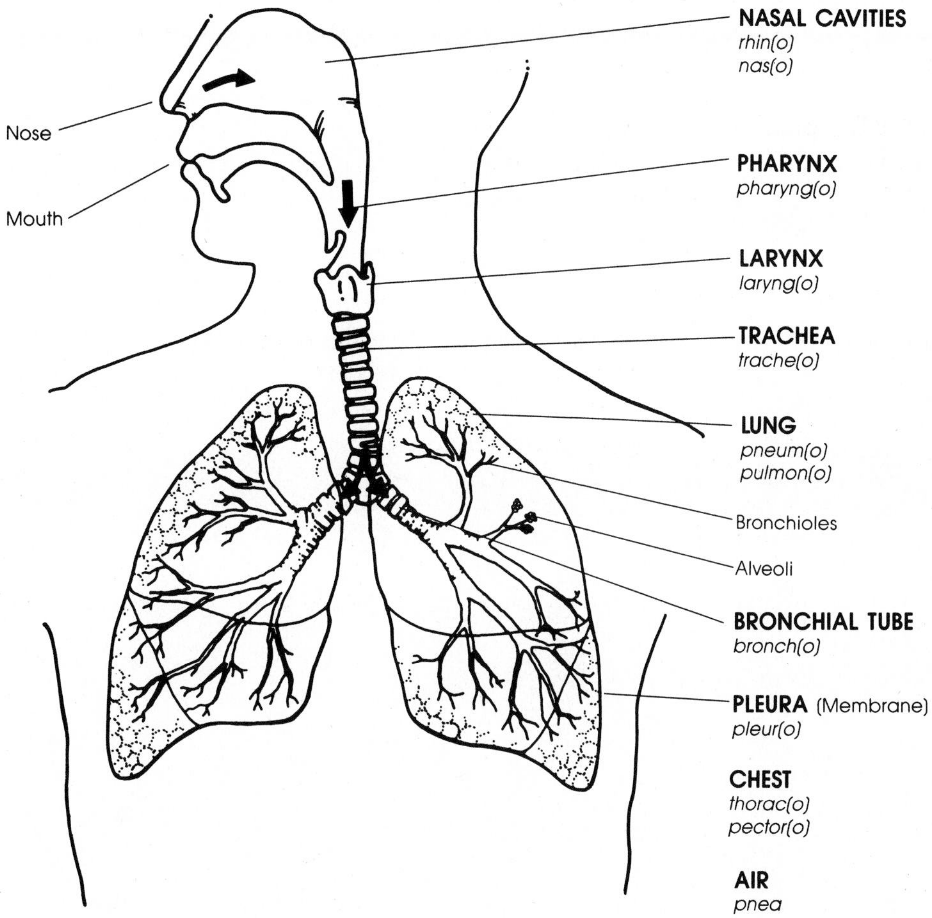

RESPIRATORY SYSTEM

Orientation

The respiratory system is a continuous open passage from the mouth and nose through the head, neck, and chest to the lungs. Breathing in and out (external respiration) allows oxygen to enter and carbon dioxide to pass from the body. The main part of the respiratory system involves the nose, mouth, pharynx, larynx, trachea, bronchi, alveoli, and lungs.

Air enters the nose through the nostrils (openings in the nose). There are numerous hairs in the nostrils which serve to filter dust and dirt from the air. The air then passes to the nasal cavities which are separated from the mouth by the palate. The air then passes to the pharynx which is also a passageway for foods and liquids to the digestive system. The larynx or voice box is situated between the pharynx and trachea (windpipe). The larynx contains a device called the epiglottis that closes during swallowing, thus keeping food out of the respiratory tract. Air is conducted from the larynx to the lungs by the trachea. The trachea divides into two branches called bronchi which then enter each lung. The bronchi then branch into increasingly smaller tubes called bronchioles that extend deep into the lungs.

The lungs are membranous sacs on either side of the chest. The right lung has three lobes (upper, middle, and lower), while the left lung has only two lobes (upper and lower). At the tips of the bronchioles are thin-walled alveolar sacs (alveoli) that are in close contact with blood capillaries. Gas exchange takes place at this point, as the red blood cells pick up inhaled oxygen to be distributed throughout the body. Breathing is accomplished by muscles around the ribs and diaphragm and is automatically controlled by the nervous system. The rate of breathing depends on the level of carbon dioxide in the bloodstream. To lessen friction between the lungs and chest cavity, the surfaces of both are lined with a membrane called the pleura.

LESSON

26

Terminology Presentation

Listen to the Lab Tape provided by your instructor, and you will hear the words presented in this lesson. Read the words as they are said, noticing spelling and pronunciation. The recording will tell you when the presentation for this lesson is completed and will give you any further instructions. Do not go on to the next recorded lesson until you have completed Lesson 26 and feel that you know the words and word parts that have been presented.

• • • ▸ *Start Audio*

thorac(o) a word element denoting the chest or thorax

WORD	WORD PART	DEFINITION	ANSWER
1. thoracocyllosis (tho′rah-ko-si-lo′sis)	-cyllosis	crippling, deformity	1. ________
2. thoracodynia (tho′rah-ko-din′e-ah)	-dynia	pain	2. ________
3. thoracentesis (tho′rah-sen-te′sis)	-centesis	surgical puncture	3. ________
4. thoracoscopy (tho′rah-kos′ko-pe)	-scopy	examine	4. ________
5. thoracomyodynia (tho′rah-ko-mi′o-din′e-ah)	my(o) -dynia	muscle pain	5. ________
6. thoracoplasty (tho′rah-ko-plas′te)	-plasty	plastic surgery	6. ________
7. thoracotomy (tho′rah-kot′o-me)	-tomy	incision, cutting into	7. ________

pnea a word ending denoting breathing or air or gas

WORD	WORD PART	DEFINITION	ANSWER
8. eupnea (up-ne′ah)	eu-	well, normal	8. ________
9. apnea (ap-ne′ah)	a-	without, lack of	9. ________

10. dyspnea (disp′ne-ah)	dys-	abnormal, painful	**10.** ________
11. orthopnea (or′thop-ne′ah)	orth(o)-	straight, normal	**11.** ________
12. oligopnea (ol′i-gop-ne′ah)	oligo-	few	**12.** ________
13. hyperpnea (hi′perp-ne′ah)	hyper-	above, over, abundant	**13.** ________
14. tachypnea (tak′ip-ne′ah)	tachy-	fast	**14.** ________

■ • • • *Stop Audio at Tone*

Study the 14 words and word parts for this lesson. Practice each word several times, checking your spelling and repeating the meaning to yourself. Listen to the recording and pronounce the words as many times as necessary. When you feel that you know the words and word parts well, you are ready to go on to the next step.

Use a sheet of paper to cover all columns except the Answer Column on the previous page. The words you have learned will be presented again on the recording. As each word is pronounced, write it in the space provided in the Answer Column.

• • • ▶ *Start Audio*

After stopping the tape player, check the words you have written against the words in the left-hand column. If any words are misspelled, practice writing them correctly. When you feel that you know and understand the words and word parts, go on to the Terminology Practice.

PRACTICE

____

____

____

____

____

____

____

____

____

Name ______________________ Date ______________ Errors ________

LESSON 26: TERMINOLOGY PRACTICE

Without looking at your previous work, write the word that is described by each definition.

thorac(o) **and *pnea***

DEFINITION	TERM
1. Pain in the muscles of the chest	______________
2. Surgical puncture or tap of the chest	______________
3. Abnormally fast rate of breathing	______________
4. Temporary absence of breathing	______________
5. Inability to breathe unless one is in an upright position	______________
6. Incision into the chest	______________
7. Retarded or small amount of breathing	______________
8. Examination of the chest	______________
9. Increase in the depth and rate of breathing	______________
10. A deformity of the chest	______________
11. Difficult breathing	______________
12. Plastic surgery on the chest	______________
13. Easy, normal breathing	______________
14. Pain in the chest region	______________

Check your answers against the word and definition lists on the first page of this lesson. If you have any errors, count them and write the number in the blank at the top of the page. Practice any missed or misspelled words on the next page. Sign your work and give it to your instructor. You are now ready for the next lesson.

PRACTICE

LESSON

27 Terminology Presentation

Listen to the Lab Tape provided by your instructor, and you will hear the words presented in this lesson. Read the words as they are said, noticing spelling and pronunciation. The recording will tell you when the presentation for this lesson is completed and will give you any further instructions. Do not go on to the next recorded lesson until you have completed Lesson 27 and feel that you know the words and word parts that have been presented.

Start Audio

trache(o) a word part indicating the trachea or windpipe

WORD	WORD PART	DEFINITION	ANSWER
1. tracheopyosis (tra′ke-o-pi-o′sis)	py(o) -osis	pus, suppuration condition, process, increase, disease	1. ______
2. tracheotomy (tra′ke-ot′o-me)	-tomy	incision, cutting into	2. ______
3. tracheoplasty (tra′ke-o-plas′te)	-plasty	plastic surgery	3. ______
4. tracheostenosis (tra′ke-o-ste-no′sis)	-stenosis	narrowing	4. ______
5. tracheopathy (tra′ke-op′ah-the)	-pathy	disease	5. ______
6. tracheorrhaphy (tra′ke-or′ah-fe)	-rrhaphy	suture, surgical repair	6. ______
7. tracheitis (tra′ke-i′tis)	-itis	inflammation	7. ______

laryng(o) a word part denoting the larynx (voice box)

WORD	WORD PART	DEFINITION	ANSWER
8. laryngitis (lar′in-ji′tis)	-itis	inflammation	8. ______

9. laryngeal (lah-rin'je-al)	-al	of, pertaining to	9. ________
10. laryngoplegia (lar'ing-go-ple'je-ah)	-plegia	paralysis	10. ________
11. laryngostenosis (lah-ring'go-ste-no'sis)	-stenosis	narrowing	11. ________
12. laryngospasm (lah-ring'go-spazm)	-spasm	contraction	12. ________
13. laryngoscope (lah-ring'go-skop)	-scope	viewing instrument	13. ________
14. laryngostomy (lar'ing-gos'to-me)	-stomy	connection, opening	14. ________
15. laryngocentesis (lah-ring'go-sen-te'sis)	-centesis	surgical puncture	15. ________

■ • • • *Stop Audio at Tone*

Study the 15 words and word parts for this lesson. Practice each word several times, checking your spelling and repeating the meaning to yourself. Listen to the recording and pronounce the words as many times as necessary. When you feel that you know the words and word parts well, you are ready to go on to the next step.

Use a sheet of paper to cover all columns except the Answer Column on the previous page. The words you have learned will be presented again on the recording. As each word is pronounced, write it in the space provided in the Answer Column.

• • • ▶ *Start Audio*

After stopping the tape player, check the words you have written against the words in the left-hand column. If any words are misspelled, practice writing them correctly. When you feel that you know and understand the words and word parts, go on to the Terminology Practice.

PRACTICE

Name ______________________ Date ______________ Errors ________

LESSON 27: TERMINOLOGY PRACTICE

Without looking at your previous work, write the word that is described by each definition.

trache(o) and *laryng(o)*

DEFINITION	TERM
1. Paralysis of the larynx	______________
2. Surgical repair or suture of the trachea	______________
3. Surgical puncture of the larynx	______________
4. Narrowing of the trachea	______________
5. Inflammation of the larynx	______________
6. Plastic surgery on the trachea	______________
7. Spasmodic closure of the larynx	______________
8. Any disease of the trachea	______________
9. The creation of an artificial opening into the larynx	______________
10. Of or pertaining to the larynx	______________
11. Narrowing of the larynx	______________
12. Suppurative inflammation of the trachea	______________
13. Incision into the trachea	______________
14. Inflammation of the trachea	______________
15. Instrument used to examine the larynx	______________

Check your answers against the word and definition lists on the first page of this lesson. If you have any errors, count them and write the number in the blank at the top of the page. Practice any missed or misspelled words on the next page. Sign your work and give it to your instructor. You are now ready for the next lesson.

PRACTICE

LESSON

28 Terminology Presentation

Listen to the Lab Tape provided by your instructor, and you will hear the words presented in this lesson. Read the words as they are said, noticing spelling and pronunciation. The recording will tell you when the presentation for this lesson is completed and will give you any further instructions. Do not go on to the next recorded lesson until you have completed Lesson 28 and feel that you know the words and word parts that have been presented.

••• ▶ *Start Audio*

bronch(o) a word part denoting the bronchi (plural) or bronchus (singular), the air passages within the lungs

WORD	WORD PART	DEFINITION	ANSWER
1. bronchorrhea (brong-ko-re'ah)	-rrhea	flow	1. ____________
2. bronchiectasis (brong'ke-ek'tah-sis)	-ectasis	dilatation, expansion	2. ____________
3. bronchitis (brong-ki'tis)	-itis	inflammation	3. ____________
4. bronchoedema (brong'ko-e-de'mah)	-edema	swelling	4. ____________
5. bronchoscopy (brong-kos'ko-pe)	-scopy	examine	5. ____________
6. bronchoplegia (brong'ko-ple'je-ah)	-plegia	paralysis	6. ____________
7. bronchopneumonitis (brong'ko-nu'mo-ni'tis)	pneum(o) -itis	lungs inflammation	7. ____________

pleur(o) a combining form indicating the pleura (the membrane lining the chest cavity and covering the lungs)

WORD	WORD PART	DEFINITION	ANSWER
8. pleural (ploor'al)	-al	of, pertaining to	8. ____________

9. pleuralgia (ploor-al'je-ah)	-algia	pain	9. ________
10. pleuroclysis (ploo-rok'li-sis)	-clysis	wash out	10. ________
11. pleurorrhea (ploor'o-re'ah)	-rrhea	flow, effusion	11. ________
12. pleurotomy (ploor-ot'o-me)	-tomy	incision, cutting	12. ________
13. pleurocentesis (ploor'o-sen-te'sis)	-centesis	surgical puncture	13. ________
14. pleurocele (ploor'o-sel)	-cele	tumor, swelling, hernia	14. ________

■ • • • *Stop Audio at Tone*

Study the 14 words and word parts for this lesson. Practice each word several times, checking your spelling and repeating the meaning to yourself. Listen to the recording and pronounce the words as many times as necessary. When you feel that you know the words and word parts well, you are ready to go on to the next step.

Use a sheet of paper to cover all columns except the Answer Column on the previous page. The words you have learned will be presented again on the recording. As each word is pronounced, write it in the space provided in the Answer Column.

• • • ▶ *Start Audio*

After stopping the tape player, check the words you have written against the words in the left-hand column. If any words are misspelled, practice writing them correctly. When you feel that you know and understand the words and word parts, go on to the Terminology Practice.

PRACTICE

____

____

____

____

____

____

____

____

Name ______________________ Date ______________ Errors ________

LESSON 28: TERMINOLOGY PRACTICE

Without looking at your previous work, write the word that is described by each definition.

bronch(o) and *pleur(o)*

DEFINITION	TERM
1. Effusion of fluid into the pleura	______________
2. Excessive secretion of mucus from the bronchial mucous membrane	______________
3. Inspection or examination of the bronchi	______________
4. Herniation of lung tissue or of the pleura	______________
5. The flushing out of the pleural cavity	______________
6. Dilatation of the bronchi	______________
7. Paralysis of the bronchi	______________
8. Surgical puncture or tap of the pleura	______________
9. Inflammation of the bronchi	______________
10. Swelling of the mucosa of the bronchi	______________
11. Incision into the pleura	______________
12. Of or relating to the pleura	______________
13. Inflammation of the lungs originating at the bronchi	______________
14. Pain in the pleural region	______________

Check your answers against the word and definition lists on the first page of this lesson. If you have any errors, count them and write the number in the blank at the top of the page. Practice any missed or misspelled words on the next page. Sign your work and give it to your instructor. You are now ready for the next lesson.

PRACTICE

LESSON

29 Terminology Presentation

Listen to the Lab Tape provided by your instructor, and you will hear the words presented in this lesson. Read the words as they are said, noticing spelling and pronunciation. The recording will tell you when the presentation for this lesson is completed and will give you any further instructions. Do not go on to the next recorded lesson until you have completed Lesson 29 and feel that you know the words and word parts that have been presented.

• • • ▶ *Start Audio*

rhin(o) a combining form denoting the nose

WORD	WORD PART	DEFINITION	ANSWER
1. rhinodynia (ri′no-din′e-ah)	-dynia	pain	1. ________
2. rhinesthesia (ri′nes-the′ze-ah)	-esthesia	perception, sense	2. ________
3. rhinolith (ri′no-lith)	-lith	stone	3. ________
4. rhinorrhagia (ri′no-ra′je-ah)	-rrhagia	excessive flow, bleeding	4. ________
5. rhinocheiloplasty (ri-no-ki′lo-plas′te)	cheil(o) -plasty	lip plastic surgery	5. ________
6. rhinitis (ri-ni′tis)	-itis	inflammation	6. ________
7. rhinomycosis (ri′no-mi-ko′sis)	mycosis	fungus	7. ________

pneumon(o), pneum(o), pneum(ato), or ***pneum(a)*** a combining form denoting the lungs, respiration, air, or gas

WORD	WORD PART	DEFINITION	ANSWER
8. pneumonitis (nu′mo-ni′tis)	-itis	inflammation	8. ________

9. pneumonography (nu′mo-nog′rah-fe)	-graphy	recording	9. ______
10. pneumomelanosis (nu′mo-mel′ah-no′sis)	melan(o) -osis	black condition, process, increase, disease	10. ______
11. pneumodynamics (nu′mo-di-nam′iks)	-dynamics	force	11. ______
12. pneumoencephalography (nu′mo-en-sef′ah-log′rah-fe)	encephal -graphy	brain recording	12. ______
13. pneumoconiosis (nu′mo-ko′ne-o′sis)	coni(o) -osis	dust disease, condition, process, increase	13. ______
14. pneumothorax (nu′mo-tho′raks)	thorax	chest	14. ______
15. pneumocentesis (nu′mo-sen-te′sis)	-centesis	surgical puncture	15. ______

■ • • • *Stop Audio at Tone*

Study the 15 words and word parts for this lesson. Practice each word several times, checking your spelling and repeating the meaning to yourself. Listen to the recording and pronounce the words as many times as necessary. When you feel that you know the words and word parts well, you are ready to go on to the next step.

Use a sheet of paper to cover all columns except the Answer Column on the previous page. The words you have learned will be presented again on the recording. As each word is pronounced, write it in the space provided in the Answer Column.

• • • ▸ *Start Audio*

After stopping the tape player, check the words you have written against the words in the left-hand column. If any words are misspelled, practice writing them correctly. When you feel that you know and understand the words and word parts, go on to the Terminology Practice.

PRACTICE

______

______

______

______

______

Name ____________________ Date ____________ Errors ________

LESSON 29: TERMINOLOGY PRACTICE

Without looking at your previous work, write the word that is described by each definition.

pneum(o) and *rhin(o)*

DEFINITION	TERM
1. The dynamics of the respiratory system	____________
2. Surgical puncture for aspiration of the lung	____________
3. Plastic surgery on the lip and nose	____________
4. Nosebleed	____________
5. X-ray of the lung	____________
6. The blackening of the lungs as from coal dust	____________
7. A stone or concretion of the nose	____________
8. Pertaining to the sense of smell	____________
9. Inflammation of the mucous membrane of the nose	____________
10. A disease caused by dust or other particulates in the lungs	____________
11. Fungus infection of the nose	____________
12. Accumulation of air in the chest cavity	____________
13. Radiographic films of the brain utilizing injections of air or gas	____________
14. Pain in the nose or nasal area	____________
15. Inflammation of the lung	____________

Check your answers against the word and definition lists on the first page of this lesson. If you have any errors, count them and write the number in the blank at the top of the page. Practice any missed or misspelled words on the next page. Sign your work and give it to your instructor. You are now ready for the next lesson.

PRACTICE

Name ______________________ Date ______________ Errors __________

LESSON 30 | TERMINOLOGY REVIEW FOR TEST 6

This is a review of the word parts you have learned in the preceding four lessons. Some of the medical terms listed below may be new, but they are made up of word parts that you have already learned.

Unlike the review for Test 5, the words are not written out for you. As each word is pronounced on the Lab Tape, write it in the appropriate numbered blank on the left.

• • • ▶ *Start Audio*

WORD	WORD PART	MEANING OF WORD PART
1. ______________	__________	______________________
	__________	______________________
	__________	______________________
2. ______________	__________	______________________
	__________	______________________
	__________	______________________
3. ______________	__________	______________________
	__________	______________________
	__________	______________________
4. ______________	__________	______________________
	__________	______________________
	__________	______________________
5. ______________	__________	______________________
	__________	______________________
	__________	______________________
6. ______________	__________	______________________
	__________	______________________
	__________	______________________
7. ______________	__________	______________________
	__________	______________________
	__________	______________________

8. ______________ ______________ ______________

______________ ______________

______________ ______________

9. ______________ ______________ ______________

______________ ______________

______________ ______________

10. ______________ ______________ ______________

______________ ______________

______________ ______________

11. ______________ ______________ ______________

______________ ______________

______________ ______________

12. ______________ ______________ ______________

______________ ______________

______________ ______________

13. ______________ ______________ ______________

______________ ______________

______________ ______________

14. ______________ ______________ ______________

______________ ______________

______________ ______________

15. ______________ ______________ ______________

______________ ______________

______________ ______________

■ • • • *Stop Audio at Tone*

After all 15 words have been written, write the word parts for each one and fill in the meanings of the parts. Use the Glossary or a dictionary to check your spellings and definitions. Practice the words on a separate sheet of paper, paying particular attention to any you missed or misspelled.

When you feel you know the words and word parts well, sign your work, indicate the number of errors, and turn your work in to your instructor.

You are now ready for the Extra Credit Review (if your instructor assigns it) or Test 6.

Name ______________________ Date ______________ Errors ________

LESSON 30 — EXTRA CREDIT REVIEW

This Extra Credit Review should be done at the discretion of your instructor. If you are instructed to complete this portion of the Review, turn your paper in to your instructor when you are finished.

PART A

Write the proper term for the following 20 definitions to the right of the given definition.

DEFINITION	TERM
1. Temporary absence of breathing	______________
2. A deformity of the chest	______________
3. The creation of an artificial opening into the larynx	______________
4. Dilatation of the bronchi	______________
5. Herniation of lung tissue or the pleura	______________
6. Surgical puncture of the larynx	______________
7. Pertaining to the sense of smell	______________
8. Plastic surgery on the lip and nose	______________
9. The blackening of a lung as from coal dust	______________
10. The flushing out of the pleural cavity	______________
11. Inability to breathe unless one is in an upright position	______________
12. Radiographic films of the brain utilizing injections of air or gas	______________
13. Pain in the nose	______________
14. Inflammation of the lungs originating at the bronchi	______________
15. Nosebleed	______________
16. Incision into the trachea	______________
17. Plastic surgery on the chest	______________

18. Difficult breathing ____________________

19. Suppurative inflammation of the trachea ____________________

20. Pain in the pleural region ____________________

PART B

Match the following definitions with the terms given. Place the correct letter of the definition to the left of the term.

TERM	DEFINITION
______ 21. laryngostenosis	a. difficult breathing
______ 22. tracheotomy	b. surgical repair or suture of the trachea
______ 23. thoracodynia	c. inflammation of the bronchi
______ 24. dyspnea	d. narrowing of the larynx
______ 25. rhinomycosis	e. fungus infection of the nose
______ 26. bronchoplegia	f. surgical procedure for aspiration of the lung
______ 27. thoracomyodynia	g. pain in the muscles of the chest
______ 28. tracheorrhaphy	h. incision into the trachea
______ 29. pneumocentesis	i. paralysis of the bronchi
______ 30. bronchitis	j. pain in the chest region

You may now go on to Test 6.

SECTION

7 Digestive System

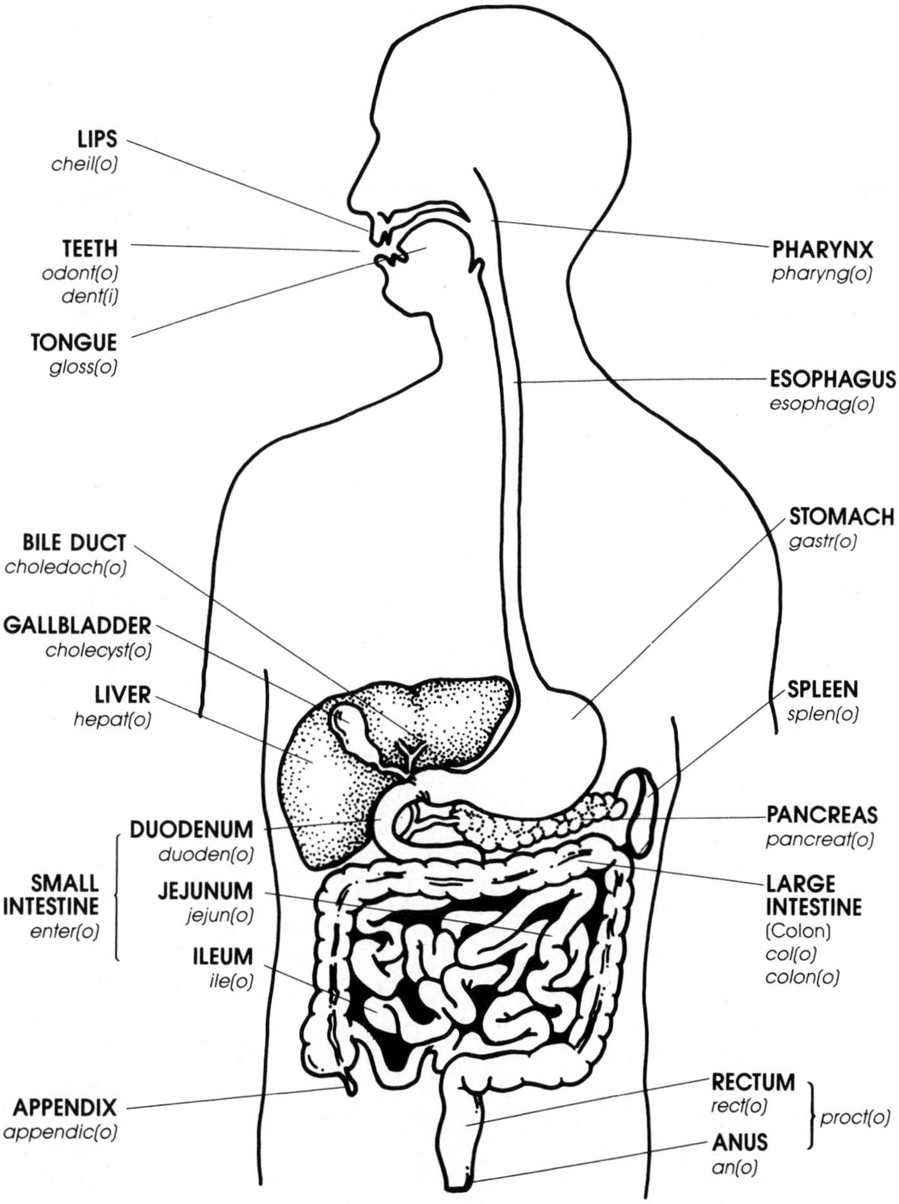

LIPS
cheil(o)
TEETH
odont(o)
dent(i)
TONGUE
gloss(o)
PHARYNX
pharyng(o)
ESOPHAGUS
esophag(o)
STOMACH
gastr(o)
BILE DUCT
choledoch(o)
GALLBLADDER
cholecyst(o)
LIVER
hepat(o)
SPLEEN
splen(o)
DUODENUM
duoden(o)
PANCREAS
pancreat(o)
SMALL INTESTINE
enter(o)
JEJUNUM
jejun(o)
ILEUM
ile(o)
LARGE INTESTINE
(Colon)
col(o)
colon(o)
APPENDIX
appendic(o)
RECTUM
rect(o)
ANUS
an(o)
proct(o)

DIGESTIVE SYSTEM

Orientation

The digestive system carries out five important functions: (a) breaking up food into smaller pieces, (b) transporting food through the alimentary or digestive tract by means of rhythmic muscular contractions (peristalsis), (c) secreting digestive enzymes, (d) promoting absorption of nutrients into the bloodstream, and (e) excreting the solid wastes of digestion.

The digestive system consists of the mouth, pharynx, esophagus, stomach, small intestine, large intestine, and secretory glands (salivary glands, liver, and pancreas), collectively referred to as the alimentary canal. Food is first broken up into smaller pieces by the teeth and mixed with saliva, a fluid that coats the pieces to make swallowing easier. It then passes through the pharynx, to and through the esophagus, which extends from the pharynx to the stomach.

The stomach has muscular valves called sphincters, which keep the food flowing in one direction. In the stomach, the food is mixed with gastric juices. These juices are composed of acids and enzymes which dissolve food, destroy bacteria, and break down meat tissue. Normally, the food is processed through the stomach in 2 to 6 hours. Food passes from the stomach to the small intestine through a valve called the pyloric sphincter.

In the first part of the small intestine, the duodenum, the nutrients are mixed with very strong digestive enzymes secreted by the accessory organs (the liver, gallbladder, and pancreas). In the remainder of the small intestine, the jejunum and ileum, nutrients are further broken down and then absorbed through the intestinal lining into the bloodstream. Unabsorbed nutrients then pass into the colon or large intestine. The pouch at the beginning of the colon is known as the cecum. Attached to the cecum is a small tube called the vermiform appendix. The four parts of the colon are the ascending, transverse, descending, and rectosigmoid segments. Here, liquid is reabsorbed into the body, so that a solid waste product (fecal material) can leave the body through the rectum and its opening, the anus.

LESSON 31

Terminology Presentation

Listen to the Lab Tape provided by your instructor, and you will hear the words presented in this lesson. Read the words as they are said, noticing spelling and pronunciation. The recording will tell you when the presentation for this lesson is completed and will give you any further instructions. Do not go on to the next recorded lesson until you have completed Lesson 31 and feel that you know the words and word parts that have been presented.

• • • ▸ *Start Audio*

proct(o) a word element denoting the rectum or anus

WORD	WORD PART	DEFINITION	ANSWER
1. proctologist (prok-tol′o-jist)	-logist	specialist	1. ______
2. proctatresia (prok′tah-tre′ze-ah)	a- -tresia	without, lack of opening, hole	2. ______
3. proctoptosis (prok′top-to′sis)	-ptosis	falling or prolapse	3. ______
4. proctocele (prok′to-sel)	-cele	tumor, swelling, hernia	4. ______
5. proctopexy (prok′to-pek′se)	-pexy	fix, fasten	5. ______
6. proctorrhea (prok′to-re′ah)	-rrhea	flow	6. ______
7. proctoscopy (prok-tos′ko-pe)	-scopy	examine	7. ______

enter(o) a word element indicating the intestines

WORD	WORD PART	DEFINITION	ANSWER
8. enterorrhagia (en′ter-o-ra′je-ah)	-rrhagia	excessive flow, bleeding	8. ______
9. enterococcus (en′ter-o-kok′us)	-coccus	bacteria	9. ______

10. enterolithiasis (en′ter-o-li-thi′ah-sis)	-lithiasis	stones	**10.** ________________
11. enterauxe (en′ter-awk′se)	-auxe	increase	**11.** ________________
12. enterorrhexis (en′ter-o-rek′sis)	-rrhexis	rupture	**12.** ________________
13. enterocleisis (en′ter-o-kli′sis)	-cleisis	closure	**13.** ________________
14. enterokinesis (en′ter-o-ki-ne′sis)	-kinesis	movement	**14.** ________________
15. enteroclysis (en′ter-ok′li-sis)	-clysis	wash out	**15.** ________________

■ • • • *Stop Audio at Tone*

Study the 15 words and word parts for this lesson. Practice each word several times, checking your spelling and repeating the meaning to yourself. Listen to the recording and pronounce the words as many times as necessary. When you feel that you know the words and word parts well, you are ready to go on to the next step.

Use a sheet of paper to cover all columns except the Answer Column on the previous page. The words you have learned will be presented again on the recording. As each word is pronounced, write it in the space provided in the Answer Column.

• • • ▸ *Start Audio*

After stopping the tape player, check the words you have written against the words in the left-hand column. If any words are misspelled, practice writing them correctly. When you feel that you know and understand the words and word parts, go on to the Terminology Practice.

PRACTICE

Name ______________________________ Date __________________ Errors __________

LESSON 31: TERMINOLOGY PRACTICE

Without looking at your previous work, write the word that is described by each definition.

proct(o) *and* ***enter(o)***

DEFINITION	TERM
1. Specialist in the diagnosis and treatment of rectal disorders	______________
2. Blockage or closure of the intestine	______________
3. Enlargement of the intestinal wall	______________
4. Hernial protrusion of the rectum	______________
5. Anal atresia, absence of a proper rectal opening	______________
6. Injection or introduction of liquid into the intestine	______________
7. Muscular movement of the intestinal canal—peristalsis	______________
8. Examination of the rectum by the use of a proctoscope	______________
9. Stones or calculi found in the intestine	______________
10. A mucoserous discharge from the rectum	______________
11. Rupture of the intestinal wall	______________
12. Prolapse or falling of the rectum	______________
13. Hemorrhage from the intestine	______________
14. A type of intestinal bacteria	______________
15. Surgical fixing or fastening of the rectum	______________

Check your answers against the word and definition lists on the first page of this lesson. If you have any errors, count them and write the number in the blank at the top of the page. Practice any missed or misspelled words in the space provided. Sign your work and give it to your instructor. You are now ready for the next lesson.

PRACTICE

LESSON

32 Terminology Presentation

Listen to the Lab Tape provided by your instructor, and you will hear the words presented in this lesson. Read the words as they are said, noticing spelling and pronunciation. The recording will tell you when the presentation for this lesson is completed and will give you any further instructions. Do not go on to the next recorded lesson until you have completed Lesson 32.

• • • ▶ *Start Audio*

hepat(o), hepat(ico) word parts denoting the liver

WORD	WORD PART	DEFINITION	ANSWER
1. hepatic (he-pat′ik)	-ic	pertaining to	1. ________
2. hepatatrophy (hep′ah-tat′ro-fe)	a- -trophy	without, lack of nourishment	2. ________
3. hepatorenal (hep′ah-to-re′nal)	ren(o) -al	kidney of, pertaining to	3. ________
4. hepatomegaly (hep′ah-to-meg′ah-le)	-megaly	enlargement	4. ________
5. hepaticolithotripsy (he-pat′i-ko-lith′o-trip-se)	lith(o) -tripsy	stone crush	5. ________
6. hepatitis (hep′ah-ti′tis)	-itis	inflammation	6. ________
7. hepatorrhaphy (hep′ah-tor′ah-fe)	-rrhaphy	suture, surgical repair	7. ________

gloss(o), gloss(ia) word parts denoting the tongue

WORD	WORD PART	DEFINITION	ANSWER
8. glossitis (glos-si′tis)	-itis	inflammation	8. ________
9. glossotrichia (glos′o-trik′e-ah)	-trich	hair or capillary vessels	9. ________

10. glossoncus (glo-song'kus)	-onc(o)	tumor	**10.** ________
11. ankyloglossia (ang'ki-lo-glos'e-ah)	ankyl(o)	bent, crooked	**11.** ________
12. glossectomy (glos-sek'to-me)	-ectomy	excision, removal	**12.** ________
13. glossodynia (glos'o-din'e-ah)	-dynia	pain	**13.** ________
14. glossorrhaphy (glo-sor'ah-fe)	-rrhaphy	suture, surgical repair	**14.** ________

■ • • • *Stop Audio at Tone*

Study the 14 words and word parts for this lesson. Practice each word several times, checking your spelling and repeating the meaning to yourself. Listen to the recording and pronounce the words as many times as necessary. When you feel that you know the words and word parts well, you are ready to go on to the next step.

Use a sheet of paper to cover all columns except the Answer Column on the previous page. The words you have learned will be presented again on the recording. As each word is pronounced, write it in the space provided in the Answer Column.

• • • ▶ *Start Audio*

After stopping the tape player, check the words you have written against the words in the left-hand column. If any words are misspelled, practice writing them correctly. When you feel that you know and understand the words and word parts, go on to the Terminology Practice.

PRACTICE

Name ______________________ Date ______________ Errors ________

LESSON 32: TERMINOLOGY PRACTICE

Without looking at your previous work, write the word that is described by each definition.

hepat(o), hepat(ico) and *gloss(o), gloss(ia)*

DEFINITION	TERM
1. A swelling or tumor of the tongue	______________
2. Surgical repair or suture of the liver	______________
3. Removal of all or part of the tongue	______________
4. Atrophy or wasting of the liver	______________
5. Hairy tongue	______________
6. Inflammation of the liver	______________
7. Enlargement of the liver	______________
8. Tongue-tied	______________
9. The operation of crushing a stone in the hepatic duct	______________
10. Pertaining to the liver and kidneys	______________
11. Inflammation of the tongue	______________
12. Pain in the tongue	______________
13. Of or pertaining to the liver	______________
14. Suture of an injured tongue	______________

Check your answers against the word and definition lists on the first page of this lesson. If you have any errors, count them and write the number in the blank at the top of the page. Practice any missed or misspelled words on the next page. Sign your work and give it to your instructor. You are now ready for the next lesson.

PRACTICE

LESSON 33

Terminology Presentation

Listen to the Lab Tape provided by your instructor, and you will hear the words presented in this lesson. Read the words as they are said, noticing spelling and pronunciation. The recording will tell you when the presentation for this lesson is completed and will give you any further instructions. Do not go on to the next recorded lesson until you have completed Lesson 33.

• • • ▸ ***Start Audio***

ile(o) a combining part denoting relationship to the ileum, the third or distal portion of the small intestine

WORD	WORD PART	DEFINITION	ANSWER
1. ileectomy (il′e-ek′to-me)	-ectomy	excision, removal	1. ____________
2. ileoproctostomy (il′e-o-prok-tos′to-me)	proct(o) -stomy	rectum connection, opening	2. ____________
3. ileorrhaphy (il′e-or′ah-fe)	-rrhaphy	suture, surgical repair	3. ____________
4. ileocecal (il′e-o-se′kal)	cec(o) -al	cecum of, pertaining to	4. ____________
5. ileotomy (il′e-ot′o-me)	-tomy	incision, cutting into	5. ____________
6. ileoentectropy (il′e-o-en-tek′tro-pe)	en ec -tropy	within out a turning	6. ____________
7. ileitis (il′e-i′tis)	-itis	inflammation	7. ____________

ili(o) a combining part denoting relationship to the ilium, the superior portion of the hip bone

WORD	WORD PART	DEFINITION	ANSWER
8. iliocostal (il′e-o-kos′tal)	cost(o) -al	rib of, pertaining to	8. ____________

9. iliac (il'e-ak)	-ac	resembling, pertaining to	9. ____________
10. iliococcygeal (il'e-o-kok-sij'e-al)	coccyg -al	coccyx of, pertaining to	10. ____________
11. iliosacral (il'e-o-sa'kral)	sacr(o) -al	sacrum of, pertaining to	11. ____________
12. iliopelvic (il'e-o-pel'vik)	pelv(i) -ic	pelvis pertaining to	12. ____________
13. iliometer (il'e-om'e-ter)	-meter	measure	13. ____________
14. iliolumbar (il'e-o-lum'ber)	lumb(o)	lumbar portion of the spine	14. ____________

■ • • • *Stop Audio at Tone*

Study the 14 words and word parts for this lesson. Practice each word several times, checking your spelling and repeating the meaning to yourself. Listen to the recording and pronounce the words as many times as necessary. When you feel that you know the words and word parts well, you are ready to go on to the next step.

Use a sheet of paper to cover all columns except the Answer Column on the previous page. The words you have learned will be presented again on the recording. As each word is pronounced, write it in the space provided in the Answer Column.

• • • ▶ *Start Audio*

After stopping the tape player, check the words you have written against the words in the left-hand column. If any words are misspelled, practice writing them correctly. When you feel that you know and understand the words and word parts, go on to the Terminology Practice.

PRACTICE

Name ______________________ Date ______________ Errors ________

LESSON 33: TERMINOLOGY PRACTICE

Without looking at your previous work, write the word that is described by each definition.

ile(o) or *ili(o)*

DEFINITION	TERM
1. An instrument for measuring the ilium	____________
2. Pertaining to the ileum and cecum	____________
3. Pertaining to the ilium	____________
4. Surgical removal or excision of the ileum	____________
5. Pertaining to the pelvis and ilium	____________
6. Pertaining to the ilium and coccyx	____________
7. Inflammation of the ileum	____________
8. Suture of the ileum	____________
9. Pertaining to the ilium and sacrum	____________
10. Making a surgical connection or opening between the ileum and rectum	____________
11. Pertaining to the ribs and ilium	____________
12. Eversion (an outward turning) of the ileum	____________
13. Incision into the ileum	____________
14. Pertaining to the lumbar and iliac region	____________

Check your answers against the word and definition lists on the first page of this lesson. If you have any errors, count them and write the number in the blank at the top of the page. Practice any missed or misspelled words on the next page. Sign your work and give it to your instructor. You are now ready for the next lesson.

PRACTICE

LESSON 34

Terminology Presentation

Listen to the Lab Tape provided by your instructor, and you will hear the words presented in this lesson. Read the words as they are said, noticing spelling and pronunciation. The recording will tell you when the presentation for this lesson is completed and will give you any further instructions. Do not go on to the next recorded lesson until you have completed Lesson 34.

• • • ▶ *Start Audio*

choledoch(o) a word part denoting bile or the common bile duct
cholecyst(o) a word part to denote the gallbladder (a bile sac)

WORD	WORD PART	DEFINITION	ANSWER
1. cholecystography (ko′le-sis-tog′rah-fe)	-graphy	recording	1. ________
2. cholecystectomy (ko′le-sis-tek′to-me)	-ectomy	excision, removal	2. ________
3. choledochotomy (ko-led′o-kot′o-me)	-tomy	incision, cutting into	3. ________
4. choledocholithotripsy (ko-led′o-ko-lith′o-trip′se)	lith(o) -tripsy	stone crush	4. ________
5. cholecystitis (ko′le-sis-ti′tis)	-itis	inflammation	5. ________
6. cholecystoptosis (ko′le-sis′to-to′sis)	-ptosis	falling	6. ________
7. choledochogastrostomy (ko-led′o-ko-gas-tros′to-me)	gastr(o) -stomy	stomach connection, opening	7. ________
8. cholelithiasis (ko′le-li-thi′ah-sis)	lith(o) -iasis	stone diseased condition	8. ________

pharyng(o) **a word part denoting the pharynx**

WORD	WORD PART	DEFINITION	ANSWER
9. pharyngonasal (fah-ring′go-na′sal)	nas(o) -al	nose of, pertaining to	9. ________

10. pharyngitis (far′in-ji′tis)	-itis	inflammation	**10.** ______
11. pharyngemphraxis (far′in-jem-frak′sis)	-emphraxis	stoppage	**11.** ______
12. pharyngoscope (fah-ring′go-skop)	-scope	viewing instrument	**12.** ______
13. pharyngostenosis (fah-ring′go-ste-no′sis)	-stenosis	narrowing	**13.** ______
14. pharyngosalpingitis (fah-ring′go-sal′pin-ji′tis)	salping(o) -itis	tube inflammation	**14.** ______
15. pharyngoxerosis (fah-ring′go-ze-ro′sis)	-xer(o) -osis	dry condition, process, increase, disease	**15.** ______

■ • • • *Stop Audio at Tone*

Study the 15 words and word parts for this lesson. Practice each word several times, checking your spelling and repeating the meaning to yourself. Listen to the recording and pronounce the words as many times as necessary. When you feel that you know the words and word parts well, you are ready to go on to the next step.

Use a sheet of paper to cover all columns except the Answer Column on the previous page. The words you have learned will be presented again on the recording. As each word is pronounced, write it in the space provided in the Answer Column.

• • • ▸ *Start Audio*

After stopping the tape player, check the words you have written against the words in the left-hand column. If any words are misspelled, practice writing them correctly. When you feel that you know and understand the words and word parts, go on to the Terminology Practice.

PRACTICE

______

______

______

______

______

______

______

Name ______________________ Date ______________ Errors ________

LESSON 34: TERMINOLOGY PRACTICE

Without looking at your previous work, write the word that is described by each definition.

choledoch(o), cholecyst(o) and *pharyng(o)*

DEFINITION	TERM
1. A downward displacement of the gallbladder	________
2. Instrument used to examine the pharynx	________
3. Inflammation of the gallbladder	________
4. The crushing of a stone in the common bile duct	________
5. Surgical connection between the stomach and common bile duct	________
6. Narrowing of the pharynx	________
7. X-ray examination of the gallbladder	________
8. Incision into the bile duct	________
9. Dryness of the pharynx	________
10. A stone in the gallbladder—gall stone	________
11. Pertaining to the nose and pharynx	________
12. Obstruction of the pharynx	________
13. Inflammation of the pharynx	________
14. Inflammation of the pharynx and eustachian tube	________
15. Excision or removal of the gallbladder	________

Check your answers against the word and definition lists on the first page of this lesson. If you have any errors, count them and write the number in the blank at the top of the page. Practice any missed or misspelled words on the next page. Sign your work and give it to your instructor. You are now ready for the next lesson.

PRACTICE

Name ______________________ Date ______________ Errors ________

LESSON 35 — TERMINOLOGY REVIEW FOR TEST 7

This is a review of the word parts you have learned in the preceding four lessons. Some of the medical terms listed below may be new, but they are made up of word parts that you have already learned. Read the words below as they are pronounced on the Lab Tape. As you listen, notice the familiar word parts which make them up.

••• ▶ *Start Audio*

WORD	WORD PART	MEANING OF WORD PART
1. proctatresia	proct	______
(prok'tah-tre'ze-ah)	-a	______
	-tresia	______
proctatresia	______	
2. ileostomy	ile(o)	______
(il'e-os'to-me)	-stomy	______
ileostomy	______	
3. glossorrhaphy	gloss(o)	______
(glo-sor'ah-fe)	-rrhaphy	______
glossorrhaphy	______	
4. hepatatrophy	hepat	______
(hep'ah-tat'ro-fe)	-a	______
	-trophy	______
hepatatrophy	______	
5. glossodynia	gloss(o)	______
(glos'o-din'e-ah)	-dynia	______
glossodynia	______	
6. cholecystogram	cholecyst(o)	______
(ko'le-sis'to-gram)	-gram	______
cholecystogram	______	
7. ileotomy	ile(o)	______
(il'e-ot'o-me)	-tomy	______
ileotomy	______	
8. iliosacral	ili(o)	______
(il'e-o-sa'kral)	sacr(o)	______
	-al	______
iliosacral	______	

9. enterorrhagia	enter(o)	______________
(en'ter-o-ra'je-ah)	-rrhagia	______________
enterorrhagia	______________	
10. proctoscopy	proct(o)	______________
(prok'tos'ko-pe)	-scopy	______________
proctoscopy	______________	
11. cholecystoptosis	cholecyst(o)	______________
(ko'le-sis'to-to'sis)	-ptosis	______________
cholecystoptosis	______________	
12. pharyngorhinitis	pharyng(o)	______________
(fah-ring'go-ri-ni'tis)	rhin(o)	______________
	-itis	______________
pharyngorhinitis	______________	
13. pharyngemphraxis	pharyng(o)	______________
(far'in-jem-frak'sis)	-emphraxis	______________
pharyngemphraxis	______________	
14. enterococcus	enter(o)	______________
(en'ter-o-kok'us)	-coccus	______________
enterococcus	______________	
15. hepatorenal	hepat(o)	______________
(hep'ah-to-re'nal)	ren(o)	______________
	-al	______________
hepatorenal	______________	

■ • • • *Stop Audio at Tone*

On the lines provided, fill in the meanings of as many of the word parts as you can from memory. Then, use the Glossary or a medical dictionary to look up any definitions you could not remember. Fill them in. On a separate piece of paper, practice writing the word parts and their meanings. Pay special attention to any which you had trouble remembering. Be sure to check your spelling.

When you have defined and reviewed all the word parts, write a definition for each whole word on the line provided. Check your definitions in a medical dictionary and make any needed corrections. Practice the words on a separate sheet of paper until you are sure that you know them. Then go on to the Extra Credit Review (if your instructor assigns it) or Test 7.

Name ______________________ Date ______________ Errors ________

LESSON 35 EXTRA CREDIT REVIEW

This Extra Credit Review should be done at the discretion of your instructor. If you are instructed to complete this portion of the Review, turn it in to your instructor when you are finished.

PART A

Each phrase below defines one of the words you have just studied. Without looking at your previous work, fill in the word that matches each definition.

DEFINITION	TERM
1. Tongue pain	______________
2. Anal atresia—absence of a proper anal opening	______________
3. A surgical opening into the ileum	______________
4. Pertaining to the liver and kidneys	______________
5. Obstruction of the pharynx	______________
6. Intestinal hemorrhage or bleeding	______________
7. X-ray examination of the gallbladder	______________
8. Incision into the ileum	______________
9. A type of intestinal bacteria	______________
10. Examination of the rectum via a proctoscope	______________
11. Atrophy or wasting of the liver	______________
12. Suture of the tongue	______________
13. Inflammation of the pharynx and nose	______________
14. Downward displacement of the gallbladder	______________
15. Pertaining to the ilium and sacrum	______________

PART B

Write the definition for the following terms to the right of the given term.

TERM	DEFINITION
16. hepaticolithotripsy	______________
17. choledochotomy	______________

18. glossoncus

19. pharyngoxerosis

20. proctologist

21. ileocecal

22. proctopexy

23. enteritis

24. cholecystitis

25. enterauxe

26. pharyngonasal

27. iliopelvic

28. hepatitis

29. iliococcygeal

30. enteroclysis

31. glossotrichia

32. ileorrhaphy

33. pharyngosalpingitis

34. ileoentectropy

35. cholelithiasis

You may now go on to Test 7.

SECTION

8 Special Senses

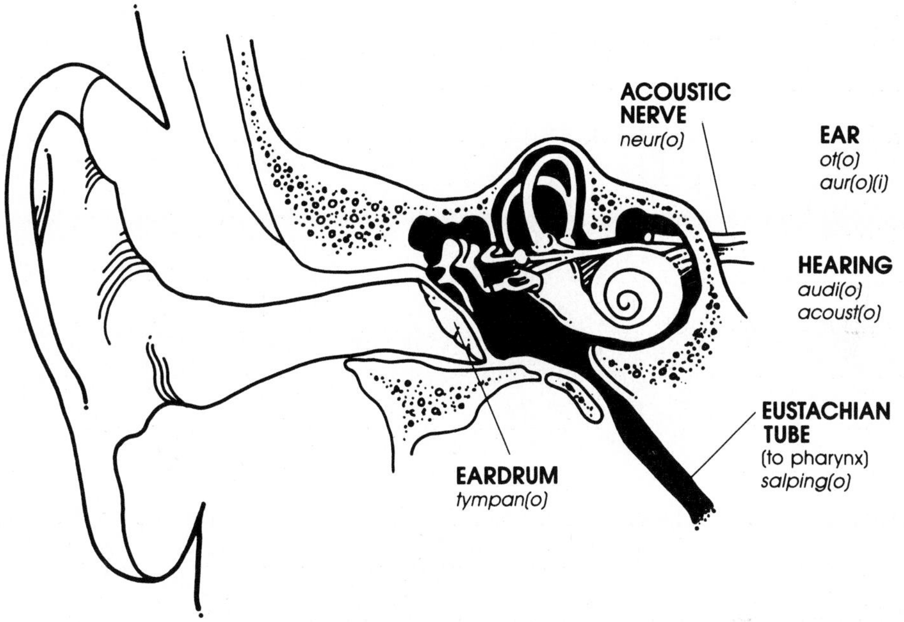
ACOUSTIC NERVE
neur(o)
EAR
ot(o)
aur(o)(i)
HEARING
audi(o)
acoust(o)
EUSTACHIAN TUBE
(to pharynx)
salping(o)
EARDRUM
tympan(o)

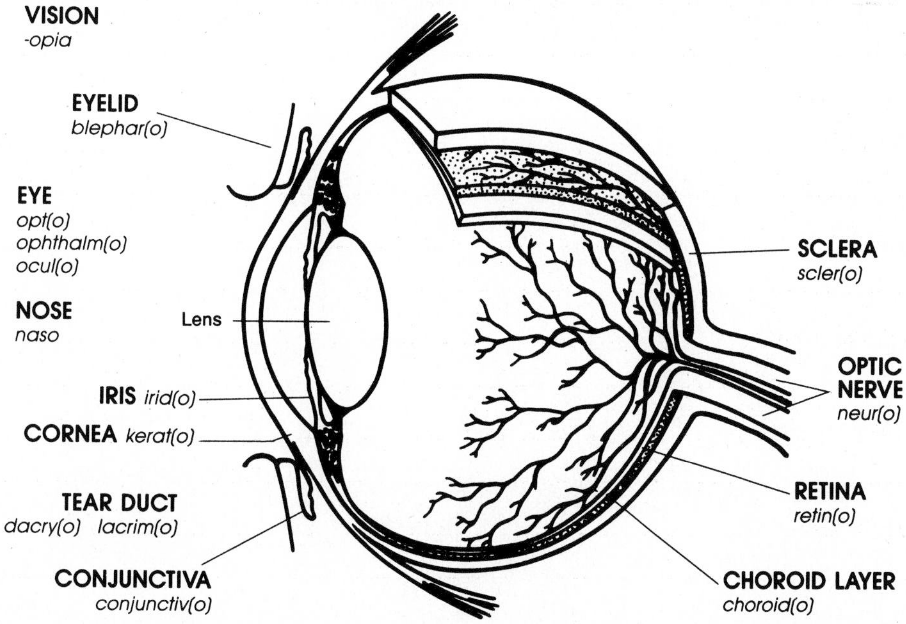
VISION
-opia
EYELID
blephar(o)
EYE
opt(o)
ophthalm(o)
ocul(o)
NOSE
naso
Lens
IRIS irid(o)
CORNEA kerat(o)
TEAR DUCT
dacry(o) lacrim(o)
CONJUNCTIVA
conjunctiv(o)
SCLERA
scler(o)
OPTIC NERVE
neur(o)
RETINA
retin(o)
CHOROID LAYER
choroid(o)

SPECIAL SENSES

Orientation

The special senses (the sensory system) are receivers of information about the environment; they allow us to feel, hear, taste, and smell. The sensory system includes the eyes, nose, ears, taste buds of the tongue, and sense receptors carried in the dermal layer of the skin.

The eye is one of the few exposed organs of the body. A system of protection is, therefore, a must for this organ. The eye is embedded in fat and is located in the bony eye orbit. It is in this orbit that the optic nerve, ocular muscles, and other vessels and nerves are attached to the eyeball. The conjunctiva, a soft membrane, covers the front part of the eyeball. The eyes are also protected by the eyelids and eyelashes, which protect the eye from dust and dirt. Tarsal glands are found in the inner part of the eyelid. These glands lubricate the edges of the eyelid. Lacrimal or tear glands keep the eyeball supplied with moisture.

The eye itself is composed of three cell layers: the sclera, the choroid layer, and the retina. The cornea, iris, pupil, and lens work together to project patterns of light upon the retina, which signals these patterns to the brain via the optic nerve.

The external ear is made up of the auricle and the external auditory meatus (ear canal). Sounds cause the eardrum to vibrate and transmit the vibrations by way of tiny bones in the inner ear to sensitive hearing cells. The inner ear is known as the labyrinth, which contains the cochlea, the semicircular canals, and the vestibule. These hearing cells signal the brain by means of the acoustic nerve.

The nasal cavity is lined with olefactory cells that convey messages of smell to the brain via the olefactory nerve. The nasal cavity is lined with a membrane that constantly secretes mucus and fluids. Foreign substances are trapped in the nasal opening by coarse and fine hairs. The glossopharyngeal nerve picks up messages from the taste buds on the tongue. The skin contains structures that are specialized to pick up the sensations of temperature, pressure, and pain.

LESSON

36 Terminology Presentation

Listen to the Lab Tape provided by your instructor, and you will hear the words presented in this lesson. Read the words as they are said, noticing spelling and pronunciation. The recording will tell you when the presentation for this lesson is completed and will give you any further instructions. Do not go on to the next recorded lesson until you have completed Lesson 36 and feel that you know the words and word parts that have been presented.

• • • ▸ *Start Audio*

ophthalm(o) a combining form denoting the eye

WORD	WORD PART	DEFINITION	ANSWER
1. ophthalmosteresis (of-thal′mo-ste-re′sis)	-steresis	privation, loss	1. ________
2. ophthalmoplegia (of-thal′mo-ple′je-ah)	-plegia	paralysis	2. ________
3. ophthalmomyitis (of-thal′mo-mi-i′tis)	my(o) -itis	muscle inflammation	3. ________
4. ophthalmology (of′thal-mol′o-je)	-logy	study of, science of	4. ________
5. ophthalmoscope (of-thal′mo-skop)	-scope	viewing instrument	5. ________
6. ophthalmodonesis (of-thal′mo-do-ne′sis)	-donesis	trembling	6. ________
7. ophthalmometer (of′thal-mom′e-ter)	-meter	measure	7. ________
8. ophthalmomalacia (of-thal′mo-mah-la′she-ah)	-malacia	softening	8. ________
9. ophthalmocopia (of-thal′mo-ko′pe-ah)	-copia	weariness, fatigue	9. ________

blephar(o) a word part denoting the eyelid			

WORD	WORD PART	DEFINITION	ANSWER
10. blepharorrhaphy (blef′ah-ror′ah-fe)	-rrhaphy	suture, surgical repair	10. ________
11. pachyblepharon (pak′e-blef′ah-ron)	pachy	thick	11. ________
12. blepharosynechia (blef′ah-ro-si-ne′ke-ah)	-synechia	a holding together	12. ________
13. blepharitis (blef′ah-ri′tis)	-itis	inflammation	13. ________
14. blepharoplasty (blef′ah-ro-plas′te)	-plasty	plastic surgery	14. ________
15. blepharoptosis (blef′ah-ro-to′sis)	-ptosis	falling	15. ________
16. blepharodiastasis (blef′ah-ro-di-as′tah-sis)	-diastasis	separation	16. ________

■ • • • *Stop Audio at Tone*

Study the 16 words and word parts for this lesson. Practice each word several times, checking your spelling and repeating the meaning to yourself. Listen to the recording and pronounce the words as many times as necessary. When you feel that you know the words and word parts well, you are ready to go on to the next step.

Use a sheet of paper to cover all columns except the Answer Column on the previous page. The words you have learned will be presented again on the recording. As each word is pronounced, write it in the space provided in the Answer Column.

• • • ▸ *Start Audio*

After stopping the tape player, check the words you have written against the words in the left-hand column. If any words are misspelled, practice writing them correctly. When you feel that you know and understand the words and word parts, go on to the Terminology Practice.

PRACTICE

____

____

____

Name ______________________ Date ______________ Errors ________

LESSON 36: TERMINOLOGY PRACTICE

Without looking at your previous work, write the word that is described by each definition.

ophthalm(o) and *blephar(o)*

DEFINITION	TERM
1. Excessive separation of the eyelids, causing the eye to open very wide	______________
2. Abnormal softness of the eye or eyeball	______________
3. Inflammation of the eyelid	______________
4. A trembling motion of the eye	______________
5. Surgical repair or suture of the eyelid	______________
6. Drooping of the eyelid	______________
7. Inflammation of the muscles that move the eyeball	______________
8. An instrument to examine the eye	______________
9. Paralysis of the eye muscle	______________
10. Eyestrain or weariness of the eye	______________
11. Thickening of the eyelid	______________
12. Loss of an eye	______________
13. Study or science of what is known of the eye and its structure	______________
14. Plastic surgery on the eyelid	______________
15. The growing together or adhesions of the eyelid	______________
16. An instrument for measuring the eye	______________

Check your answers against the word and definition lists on the first page of this lesson. If you have any errors, count them and write the number in the blank at the top of the page. Practice any missed or misspelled words in the space provided. Sign your work and give it to your instructor. You are now ready for the next lesson.

PRACTICE

LESSON

37 Terminology Presentation

Listen to the Lab Tape provided by your instructor, and you will hear the words presented in this lesson. Read the words as they are said, noticing spelling and pronunciation. The recording will tell you when the presentation for this lesson is completed and will give you any further instructions. Do not go on to the next recorded lesson until you have completed Lesson 37 and feel that you know the words and word parts that have been presented.

• • • ▶ *Start Audio*

dips(o), dips(ia) word parts denoting thirst

WORD	WORD PART	DEFINITION	ANSWER
1. dipsomania (dip'so-ma'ne-ah)	-mania	compulsion	1. ________
2. polydipsia (pol'e-dip'se-ah)	poly	much	2. ________
3. dipsotherapy (dip'so-ther'ah-pe)	-therapy	treatment	3. ________
4. dipsogen (dip'so-jen)	-gen	to produce	4. ________
5. dipsosis (dip-so'sis)	-osis	condition, process, increase, disease	5. ________

kerat(o) a combining form denoting the cornea of the eye or horny tissue

WORD	WORD PART	DEFINITION	ANSWER
6. keratectasia (ker'ah-tek-ta'ze-ah)	-ectasia	dilatation, expansion	6. ________
7. keratomycosis (ker'ah-to-mi-ko'sis)	-mycosis	fungus	7. ________
8. keratoiritis (ker'ah-to-i-ri'tis)	iri(o) -itis	iris inflammation	8. ________
9. keratocentesis (ker'ah-to-sen-te'sis)	-centesis	surgical puncture	9. ________

10. keratohelcosis (ker'ah-to-hel-ko'sis)	-helcosis	ulceration	10. ______
11. keratoplasty (ker'ah-to-plas'te)	-plasty	plastic surgery	11. ______
12. keratocele (ker'ah-to-sel')	-cele	tumor, swelling, hernia	12. ______

■ • • • *Stop Audio at Tone*

Study the 12 words and word parts for this lesson. Practice each word several times, checking your spelling and repeating the meaning to yourself. Listen to the recording and pronounce the words as many times as necessary. When you feel that you know the words and word parts well, you are ready to go on to the next step.

Use a sheet of paper to cover all columns except the Answer Column on the previous page. The words you have learned will be presented again on the recording. As each word is pronounced, write it in the space provided in the Answer Column.

• • • ▶ *Start Audio*

After stopping the tape player, check the words you have written against the words in the left-hand column. If any words are misspelled, practice writing them correctly. When you feel that you know and understand the words and word parts, go on to the Terminology Practice.

PRACTICE

Name ______________________ Date ______________ Errors ________

LESSON 37: TERMINOLOGY PRACTICE

Without looking at your previous work, write the word that is described by each definition.

dips(o), *dips(ia)* and *kerat(o)*

DEFINITION	TERM
1. Herniation of a part of the cornea	______________
2. Compulsion or uncontrollable desire to drink spiritous liquor	______________
3. Ulceration of the cornea	______________
4. Treatment by limitation of amount of water ingested	______________
5. Plastic surgery on the cornea	______________
6. Inflammation of the cornea and iris	______________
7. Protrusion of the cornea	______________
8. A condition producing thirst	______________
9. Surgical puncture of the cornea	______________
10. An agent which produces thirst	______________
11. Excessive thirst	______________
12. Fungus infection of the cornea	______________

Check your answers against the word and definition lists on the first page of this lesson. If you have any errors, count them and write the number in the blank at the top of the page. Practice any missed or misspelled words on the next page. Sign your work and give it to your instructor. You are now ready for the next lesson.

PRACTICE

LESSON 38

Terminology Presentation

Listen to the Lab Tape provided by your instructor, and you will hear the words presented in this lesson. Read the words as they are said, noticing spelling and pronunciation. The recording will tell you when the presentation for this lesson is completed and will give you any further instructions. Do not go on to the next recorded lesson until you have completed Lesson 38 and feel that you know the words and word parts that have been presented.

• • • ▶ ***Start Audio***

nas(o) a combining form to denote the nose

WORD	WORD PART	DEFINITION	ANSWER
1. nasolabial (na′zo-la′be-al)	lab(i) -al	lip of, pertaining to	1. ________
2. nasopharyngoscope (na′zo-fah-rin′go-skop)	pharyng(o) -scope	pharynx viewing instrument	2. ________
3. nasoseptal (na′zo-sep′tal)	septal	septum (a wall)	3. ________
4. nasoscope (na′zo-skop)	-scope	viewing instrument	4. ________
5. nasograph (na′zo-graf)	-graph	an instrument for recording	5. ________
6. nasal (na′zal)	-al	of, pertaining to	6. ________

ot(o) a combining form indicating the ear

WORD	WORD PART	DEFINITION	ANSWER
7. otitis (o-ti′tis)	-itis	inflammation	7. ________
8. otalgia (o-tal′je-ah)	-algia	pain	8. ________
9. otoblennorrhea (o′to-blen′o-re′ah)	-blenn(o) -rrhea	mucus flow	9. ________

10. otologist (o-tol′o-jist)	-logist	specialist	**10.** ________
11. otorrhea (o′to-re′ah)	-rrhea	flow	**11.** ________
12. otomycosis (o′to-mi-ko′sis)	-mycosis	fungus	**12.** ________
13. otopyosis (o′to-pi-o′sis)	py(o) -osis	pus, suppuration condition, process, increase, disease	**13.** ________
14. otosclerosis (o′to-skle-ro′sis)	-sclerosis	hardening	**14.** ________

■ • • • *Stop Audio at Tone*

Study the 14 words and word parts for this lesson. Practice each word several times, checking your spelling and repeating the meaning to yourself. Listen to the recording and pronounce the words as many times as necessary. When you feel that you know the words and word parts well, you are ready to go on to the next step.

Use a sheet of paper to cover all columns except the Answer Column on the previous page. The words you have learned will be presented again on the recording. As each word is pronounced, write it in the space provided in the Answer Column.

• • • ▶ *Start Audio*

After stopping the tape player, check the words you have written against the words in the left-hand column. If any words are misspelled, practice writing them correctly. When you feel that you know and understand the words and word parts, go on to the Terminology Practice.

PRACTICE

Name ______________________ Date ______________ Errors ________

LESSON 38: TERMINOLOGY PRACTICE

Without looking at your previous work, write the word that is described by each definition.

nas(o) and *ot(o)*

DEFINITION	TERM
1. A new formation of spongy bone in the ear	______
2. Inflammation of the ear	______
3. Pertaining to the nasal septum	______
4. An instrument for examination of the nasopharynx	______
5. A discharge from the ear	______
6. Pertaining to the nose and lip	______
7. Fungus infection of the ear canal	______
8. An instrument for measuring the nose	______
9. Specialist in treating ear disorders	______
10. Mucus discharge from the ear	______
11. A lighted instrument to examine the nose	______
12. Formation of pus in the ear	______
13. Pertaining to the nose	______
14. Earache or ear pain	______

Check your answers against the word and definition lists on the first page of this lesson. If you have any errors, count them and write the number in the blank at the top of the page. Practice any missed or misspelled words on the next page. Sign your work and give it to your instructor. You are now ready for the next lesson.

PRACTICE

LESSON

39 Terminology Presentation

Listen to the Lab Tape provided by your instructor, and you will hear the words presented in this lesson. Read the words as they are said, noticing spelling and pronunciation. The recording will tell you when the presentation for this lesson is completed and will give you any further instructions. Do not go on to the next recorded lesson until you have completed Lesson 39 and feel that you know the words and word parts that have been presented.

••• ▶ *Start Audio*

irid(o) a combining form denoting a relationship to the iris of the eye

WORD	WORD PART	DEFINITION	ANSWER
1. iridauxesis (ir′id-awk-se′sis)	-auxesis	increase, enlargement	1. ________
2. iridectasis (ir′i-dek′tah-sis)	-ectasis	dilatation, expansion	2. ________
3. iridomalacia (ir′i-do-mah-la′she-ah)	-malacia	softening	3. ________
4. iridosteresis (ir′i-do-ste-re′sis)	-steresis	privation, loss	4. ________
5. iridotomy (ir′i-dot′o-me)	-tomy	incision, cutting into	5. ________
6. iritis (i-ri′tis)	-itis	inflammation	6. ________
7. iridoplegia (ir′i-do-ple′je-ah)	-plegia	paralysis	7. ________

dacry(o) a combining form denoting tears or lacrimal (tear) glands or ducts

WORD	WORD PART	DEFINITION	ANSWER
8. dacryoadenitis (dak′re-o-ad′e-ni′tis)	aden(o) -itis	glands inflammation	8. ________

9. dacryoma (dak're-o'mah)	-oma	tumor	9. ______
10. dacryostenosis (dak're-o-ste-no'sis)	-stenosis	narrowing	10. ______
11. dacryolithiasis (dak're-o-li-thi'ah-sis)	-lithiasis	stone	11. ______
12. dacryocyst (dak're-o-sist')	-cyst(o)	sac	12. ______
13. dacryocystitis (dak're-o-sis-ti'tis)	-cyst(o) -itis	sac, inflammation	13. ______
14. dacryorrhea (dak're-o-re'ah)	-rrhea	flow	14. ______

■ • • • *Stop Audio at Tone*

Study the 14 words and word parts for this lesson. Practice each word several times, checking your spelling and repeating the meaning to yourself. Listen to the recording and pronounce the words as many times as necessary. When you feel that you know the words and word parts well, you are ready to go on to the next step.

Use a sheet of paper to cover all columns except the Answer Column on the previous page. The words you have learned will be presented again on the recording. As each word is pronounced, write it in the space provided in the Answer Column.

• • • ▶ *Start Audio*

After stopping the tape player, check the words you have written against the words in the left-hand column. If any words are misspelled, practice writing them correctly. When you feel that you know and understand the words and word parts, go on to the Terminology Practice.

PRACTICE

______

______

______

______

______

______

______

______

Name ______________________ Date ______________ Errors ________

LESSON 39: TERMINOLOGY PRACTICE

Without looking at your previous work, write the word that is described by each definition.

irid(o) and *dacry(o)*

DEFINITION	TERM
1. Narrowing of the lacrimal (tear) duct	________________
2. Paralysis of the iris	________________
3. Enlargement or thickening of the iris	________________
4. Inflammation of the lacrimal (tear) gland	________________
5. Inflammation of the iris	________________
6. A tumor of the lacrimal apparatus	________________
7. A lacrimal or tear sac	________________
8. Loss or absence of all or a part of the iris	________________
9. Incision into the iris	________________
10. A stone or concretion in a lacrimal gland or duct	________________
11. Dilatation of the iris	________________
12. Inflammation of the tear or lacrimal sac	________________
13. Excessive discharge of tears	________________
14. Softening of the iris	________________

Check your answers against the word and definition lists on the first page of this lesson. If you have any errors, count them and write the number in the blank at the top of the page. Practice any missed or misspelled words on the next page. Sign your work and give it to your instructor. You are now ready for the next lesson.

PRACTICE

Name ______________________ Date ______________ Errors ________

LESSON 40 | TERMINOLOGY REVIEW FOR TEST 8

This is a review of the word parts you have learned in the preceding four lessons. Some of the medical terms listed below may be new, but they are made up of word parts that you have already learned.

Unlike the review for Test 7, the words are not written out for you. As each word is pronounced on the Lab Tape, write it in the appropriate numbered blank on the left.

• • • ▸ *Start Audio*

WORD	WORD PART	MEANING OF WORD PART
1. ______________	______________	______________________
	______________	______________________
	______________	______________________
2. ______________	______________	______________________
	______________	______________________
	______________	______________________
3. ______________	______________	______________________
	______________	______________________
	______________	______________________
4. ______________	______________	______________________
	______________	______________________
	______________	______________________
5. ______________	______________	______________________
	______________	______________________
	______________	______________________
6. ______________	______________	______________________
	______________	______________________
	______________	______________________
7. ______________	______________	______________________
	______________	______________________
	______________	______________________

8. ______________ ______________ ______________

9. ______________ ______________ ______________

10. ______________ ______________ ______________

11. ______________ ______________ ______________

12. ______________ ______________ ______________

13. ______________ ______________ ______________

14. ______________ ______________ ______________

15. ______________ ______________ ______________

■ • • • *Stop Audio at Tone*

After all 15 words have been written, write the word parts for each one and fill in the meanings of the parts. Use the Glossary or a dictionary to check your spellings and definitions. Practice the words on a separate sheet of paper, paying particular attention to any you missed or misspelled.

When you feel you know the words and word parts well, sign your work, indicate the number of errors, and turn your work in to your instructor.

You are now ready for the Extra Credit Review (if your instructor assigns it) or Test 8.

Name ______________________ Date ______________ Errors ________

LESSON 40 EXTRA CREDIT REVIEW

This Extra Credit Review should be done at the discretion of your instructor. If you are instructed to complete this portion of the Review, turn your paper in to your instructor when you are finished.

PART A

Match the following terms with the definitions given. Place the correct letter of the term to the left of the definition.

DEFINITION

______ 1. Thickening of the eyelid

______ 2. Ulceration of the cornea

______ 3. Formation of pus in the ear

______ 4. A stone or concretion in the lacrimal gland or duct

______ 5. Eyestrain or weariness of the eyes

______ 6. Abnormal softening of the eye or eyeball

______ 7. Suture or surgical repair of the eyelid

______ 8. A new formation of spongy bone in the ear

______ 9. Compulsion or uncontrollable desire to drink spiritous liquor

______ 10. Paralysis of the iris

TERM

a. ophthalmocopia
b. blepharorrhaphy
c. otosclerosis
d. dipsomania
e. pachyblepharon
f. keratohelcosis
g. dacryolithiasis
h. otopyosis
i. iridoplegia
j. ophthalmomalacia

PART B

Write the definitions for the following terms to the right of the given term.

TERM	DEFINITION
11. blepharosynechia	______________________
12. keratoiritis	______________________
13. ophthalmodonesis	______________________
14. nasolabial	______________________
15. dacryocystitis	______________________

16. blepharodiastasis ______________________________

17. iridauxesis ______________________________

18. ophthalmosteresis ______________________________

19. keratoplasty ______________________________

20. iridectasis ______________________________

21. polydipsia ______________________________

22. otitis ______________________________

23. dacryostenosis ______________________________

24. otomycosis ______________________________

25. otorrhea ______________________________

You may now go on to Test 8.

SECTION

9 Endocrine System

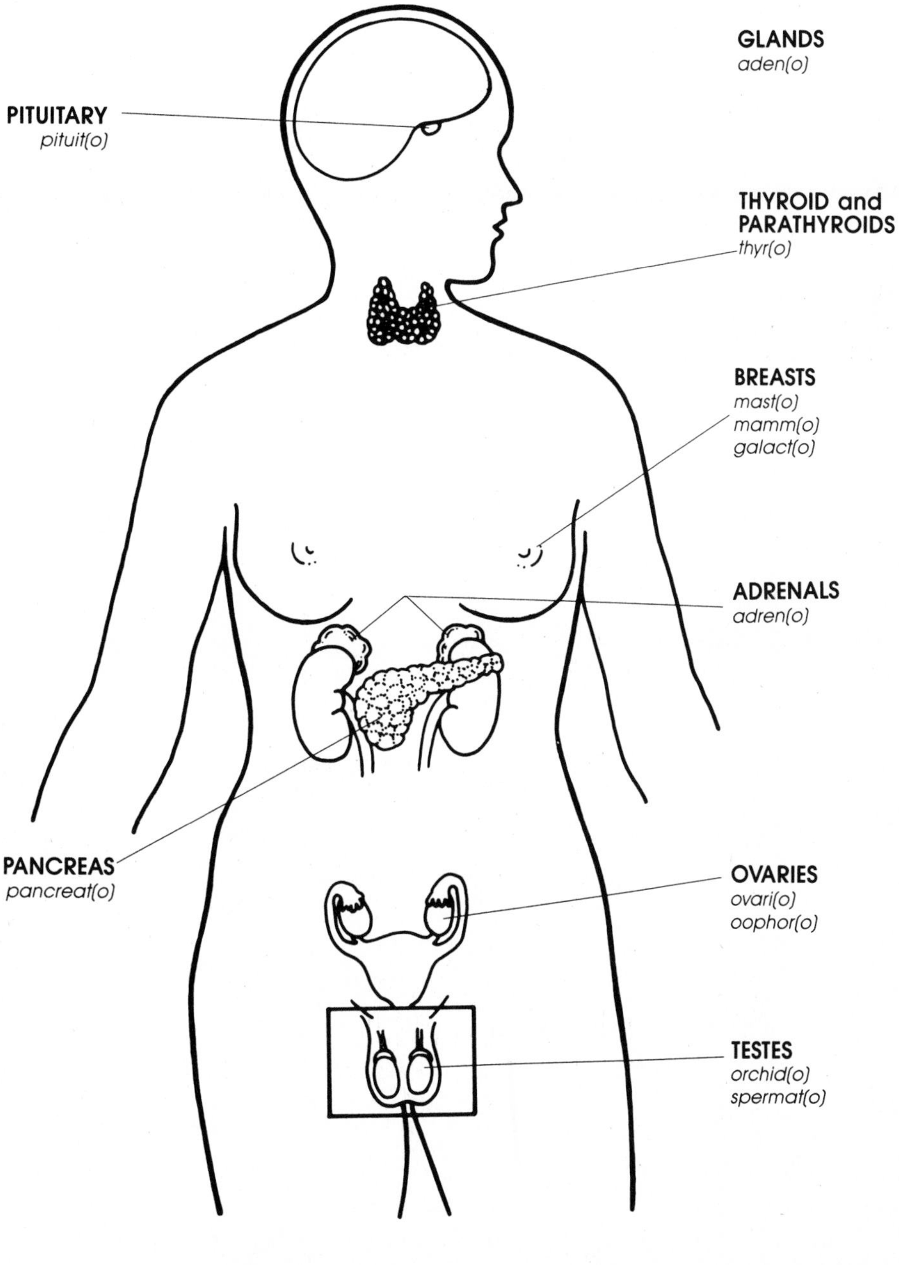

ENDOCRINE SYSTEM

Orientation

The endocrine system is made up of glands. Glands are specialized tissues that secrete chemical substances, called hormones, which help to control various body processes. Each gland produces a different hormone or hormones, and each hormone has a unique function.

The pituitary gland, also called the hypophysis, is located in the brain. It produces hormones that direct the operation of other glands, so it is sometimes referred to as the "master gland." It also produces somatotropin, which controls body growth. In females, it secretes prolactin, which stimulates glands in the breast to produce milk. The thyroid, the largest endocrine gland, produces the hormone thyroxine, which regulates metabolism, the consumption of nutrients by cells to create energy. Four small parathyroid glands, located behind the thyroid, produce a hormone that controls the body's calcium content. The thyroid is anatomically located in the neck just below the larynx.

Two adrenal glands sit atop the kidneys and produce two important sets of hormones. One set, the corticosteroids, regulate the use of proteins and sugars by the cells and the reabsorption of salt and fluids in the kidneys. The other set, epinephrine and norepinephrine, permit the body to adapt to stressful situations and emergencies by adjusting the heartbeat, respiration rate, and blood pressure. The hormones produced by these glands are stimulated by adrenocorticotropic hormone (ACTH) from the pituitary gland.

The pancreas, which is located behind the stomach, contains small groups of cells called islets of Langerhans which secrete the hormone insulin. Insulin is necessary for sugar to be metabolized and used by body tissues. The deficiency of insulin causes the disease diabetes mellitus.

Two other glands, the ovaries and testes are called the gonads and are part of the male and female reproductive systems. They secrete hormones that cause the development of secondary sex characteristics and the male and female sex cells.

LESSON

41 Terminology Presentation

Listen to the Lab Tape provided by your instructor, and you will hear the words presented in this lesson. Read the words as they are said, noticing spelling and pronunciation. The recording will tell you when the presentation for this lesson is completed and will give you any further instructions. Do not go on to the next recorded lesson until you have completed Lesson 41 and feel that you know the words and word parts that have been presented.

••• ▸ *Start Audio*

aden(o) a word element denoting the glands

WORD	WORD PART	DEFINITION	ANSWER
1. adenocarcinoma (ad′e-no-kar′si-no′mah)	-carcinoma	cancer	1. ________
2. adenitis (ad′e-ni′tis)	-itis	inflammation	2. ________
3. adenoblast (ad′e-no-blast′)	-blast	immature cell	3. ________
4. adenohypersthenia (ad′e-no-hi′per-sthe′ne-ah)	hyper	above, over, abundant	4. ________
	-sthenia	strength	
5. adenoid (ad′e-noid)	-oid	like, resembling	5. ________
6. adenoma (ad′e-no′mah)	-oma	tumor	6. ________
7. adenodynia (ad′e-no-din′e-ah)	-dynia	pain	7. ________
8. adenemphraxis (ad′e-nem-frak′sis)	-emphraxis	stoppage	8. ________

myx(o) a combining form denoting mucus or mucous membrane

	WORD	WORD PART	DEFINITION	ANSWER
9.	myxadenoma (miks'ad-e-no'mah)	aden(o) -oma	gland tumor	9. ______
10.	myxocystitis (mik'so-sis-ti'tis)	cyst(o) -itis	sac, bladder inflammation	10. ______
11.	myxoid (mik'soid)	-oid	like, resembling	11. ______
12.	myxedema (mik'se-de'mah)	-edema	swelling	12. ______
13.	myxorrhea (mik'so-re'ah)	-rrhea	flow	13. ______
14.	myxopoiesis (mik'so-poi-e'sis)	-poiesis	form, formation	14. ______

■ • • • *Stop Audio at Tone*

Study the 14 words and word parts for this lesson. Practice each word several times, checking your spelling and repeating the meaning to yourself. Listen to the recording and pronounce the words as many times as necessary. When you feel that you know the words and word parts well, you are ready to go on to the next step.

Use a sheet of paper to cover all columns except the Answer Column on the previous page. The words you have learned will be presented again on the recording. As each word is pronounced, write it in the space provided in the Answer Column.

• • • ▸ *Start Audio*

After stopping the tape player, check the words you have written against the words in the left-hand column. If any words are misspelled, practice writing them correctly. When you feel that you know and understand the words and word parts, go on to the Terminology Practice.

PRACTICE

______

______

______

______

______

Name ______________________ Date ______________ Errors ________

LESSON 41: TERMINOLOGY PRACTICE

Without looking at your previous work, write the word that is described by each definition.

aden(o) *or* ***myx(o)***

DEFINITION	TERM
1. Excessive glandular activity	______________
2. Swelling due to mucus in the tissue	______________
3. Pain in a gland	______________
4. A flow of mucus	______________
5. An embryonic cell producing glandular tissue	______________
6. Glandular cancer or carcinoma	______________
7. Inflammation of the mucous membrane of the bladder	______________
8. Like or resembling a gland or the glands	______________
9. A tumor with the structure of the mucous gland	______________
10. Making or producing mucus	______________
11. Glandular obstruction	______________
12. Inflammation of a gland or glands	______________
13. Like or resembling mucus	______________
14. A benign tumor of a gland	______________

Check your answers against the word and definition lists on the first page of this lesson. If you have any errors, count them and write the number in the blank at the top of the page. Practice any missed or misspelled words on the next page. Sign your work and give it to your instructor. You are now ready for the next lesson.

PRACTICE

LESSON 42

Terminology Presentation

Listen to the Lab Tape provided by your instructor, and you will hear the words presented in this lesson. Read the words as they are said, noticing spelling and pronunciation. The recording will tell you when the presentation for this lesson is completed and will give you any further instructions. Do not go on to the next recorded lesson until you have completed Lesson 42 and feel that you know the words and word parts that have been presented.

Start Audio

galact(o) a combining form denoting milk or a resemblance to milk

WORD	WORD PART	DEFINITION	ANSWER
1. galactogenous (gal′ak-toj′e-nus)	-genous	to produce	1. ________
2. galactophoritis (gah-lak′to-fo-ri′tis)	-phor -itis	carrying, a duct inflammation	2. ________
3. galactophlysis (gal′ak-tof′li-sis)	-phlysis	an eruption	3. ________
4. galactopoiesis (gah-lak′to-poi-e′sis)	-poiesis	form, formation	4. ________
5. galactorrhea (gah-lak′to-re′ah)	-rrhea	flow	5. ________
6. galactacrasia (gal′ak-tah-kra′se-ah)	-acrasia	a bad or abnormal mixture	6. ________
7. galactostasis (gal′ak-tos′tah-sis)	-stasis	stop	7. ________

adren(o) a combining form denoting the adrenal glands which secrete the hormone epinephrine (adrenalin, ad = near + renal = kidney)

WORD	WORD PART	DEFINITION	ANSWER
8. adrenomegaly (ad-ren′o-meg′ah-le)	-megaly	enlargement	8. ________
9. adrenalinuria (ah-dren′ah-lin-u′re-ah)	-uria	urine	9. ________

10. adrenopathy (ad'ren-op'ah-the)	-pathy	disease	10. ________
11. adrenalectomy (ah-dre'nal-ek'to-me)	-ectomy	excision, removal	11. ________
12. adrenalitis (ah-dre'nal-i'tis)	-itis	inflammation	12. ________
13. adrenoprival (ad-ren'o-pri'val)	-priv -al	to deprive of, pertaining to	13. ________
14. adrenotoxin (ad-ren'o-tok'sin)	-toxin	poison	14. ________
15. adrenokinetic (ad-re'no-ki-net'ik)	-kinetic	movement	15. ________

■ • • • *Stop Audio at Tone*

Study the 15 words and word parts for this lesson. Practice each word several times, checking your spelling and repeating the meaning to yourself. Listen to the recording and pronounce the words as many times as necessary. When you feel that you know the words and word parts well, you are ready to go on to the next step.

Use a sheet of paper to cover all columns except the Answer Column on the previous page. The words you have learned will be presented again on the recording. As each word is pronounced, write it in the space provided in the Answer Column.

• • • ▶ *Start Audio*

After stopping the tape player, check the words you have written against the words in the left-hand column. If any words are misspelled, practice writing them correctly. When you feel that you know and understand the words and word parts, go on to the Terminology Practice.

PRACTICE

____

____

____

____

____

____

____

____

Name ______________________________ Date __________________ Errors _________

LESSON 42: TERMINOLOGY PRACTICE

Without looking at your previous work, write the word that is described by each definition.

galact(o) and *adren(o)*

DEFINITION	TERM
1. Inflammation of the adrenal glands	____________
2. The presence of epinephrine in the urine	____________
3. Production of milk by the mammary glands	____________
4. Enlargement of the adrenal gland	____________
5. Producing milk	____________
6. Inflammation of the milk ducts	____________
7. Surgical removal of the adrenal gland	____________
8. Pertaining to the loss or deprivation of adrenal function	____________
9. Halting or stoppage of milk secretion	____________
10. A vesicular eruption containing a milky fluid	____________
11. Any disease of the adrenal gland	____________
12. Stimulating the adrenal gland	____________
13. Abnormal composition of mother's milk	____________
14. Excessive or spontaneous flow of milk	____________
15. Toxic or poisonous to the adrenal glands	____________

Check your answers against the word and definition lists on the first page of this lesson. If you have any errors, count them and write the number in the blank at the top of the page. Practice any missed or misspelled words on the next page. Sign your work and give it to your instructor. You are now ready for the next lesson.

PRACTICE

LESSON

43

Terminology Presentation

Listen to the Lab Tape provided by your instructor, and you will hear the words presented in this lesson. Read the words as they are said, noticing spelling and pronunciation. The recording will tell you when the presentation for this lesson is completed and will give you any further instructions. Do not go on to the next recorded lesson until you have completed Lesson 43 and feel that you know the words and word parts that have been presented.

• • • ▸ *Start Audio*

pancreat(o) a combining form denoting relationship to the pancreas

WORD	WORD PART	DEFINITION	ANSWER
1. pancreatitis (pan'kre-ah-ti'tis)	-itis	inflammation	1. ____________
2. pancreatopathy (pan'kre-ah-top'ah-the)	-pathy	disease	2. ____________
3. pancreatoid (pan-kre'ah-toid)	-oid	like, resembling	3. ____________
4. pancreatic (pan'kre-at'ik)	-ic	pertaining to	4. ____________
5. pancreathelcosis (pan'kre-ath'el-ko'sis)	-helcosis	ulceration	5. ____________
6. pancreatectomy (pan'kre-ah-tek'to-me)	-ectomy	excision, removal	6. ____________
7. pancreolysis (pan'kre-ol'i-sis)	-lysis	dissolve, break down	7. ____________
8. pancreatolith (pan'kre-at'o-lith)	-lith	stone	8. ____________

thyr(o) a combining form denoting the thyroid gland

WORD	WORD PART	DEFINITION	ANSWER
9. thyrocele (thi'ro-sel)	-cele	tumor, swelling, hernia	9. ____________

10. thyropenia (thi'ro-pe'ne-ah)	-penia	decrease	**10.** ________
11. thyroptosis (thi'rop-to'sis)	-ptosis	falling	**11.** ________
12. thyroiditis (thi'roi-di'tis)	-itis	inflammation	**12.** ________
13. thyrogenous (thi-roj'e-nus)	-genous	to produce	**13.** ________
14. thyrotoxicosis (thi'ro-tok'si-ko'sis)	-toxic -osis	poison condition, process, increase, disease	**14.** ________
15. hypothyroidism (hi'po-thi'roid-izm)	hyp(o) -ism	under, deficient condition	**15.** ________

■ • • • *Stop Audio at Tone*

Study the 15 words and word parts for this lesson. Practice each word several times, checking your spelling and repeating the meaning to yourself. Listen to the recording and pronounce the words as many times as necessary. When you feel that you know the words and word parts well, you are ready to go on to the next step.

Use a sheet of paper to cover all columns except the Answer Column on the previous page. The words you have learned will be presented again on the recording. As each word is pronounced, write it in the space provided in the Answer Column.

• • • ▸ *Start Audio*

After stopping the tape player, check the words you have written against the words in the left-hand column. If any words are misspelled, practice writing them correctly. When you feel that you know and understand the words and word parts, go on to the Terminology Practice.

PRACTICE

Name ______________________ Date ______________ Errors ________

LESSON 43: TERMINOLOGY PRACTICE

Without looking at your previous work, write the word that is described by each definition.

pancreat(o) and *thyr(o)*

DEFINITION	TERM
1. Ulceration of the pancreas	______________
2. Pertaining to the pancreas	______________
3. Deficiency of thyroid secretion	______________
4. Destruction of the pancreatic tissue	______________
5. A stone or calculi in the pancreas	______________
6. A tumor of the thyroid gland; a goiter	______________
7. Originating in the thyroid gland	______________
8. Inflammation of the pancreas	______________
9. A disease of the pancreas	______________
10. Decreased or deficient activity of the thyroid	______________
11. A disease (toxic) resulting from overactivity of the thyroid gland	______________
12. Surgical removal of the pancreas	______________
13. Downward displacement of the thyroid gland	______________
14. Inflammation of the thyroid gland	______________
15. Like or resembling the pancreas	______________

Check your answers against the word and definition lists on the first page of this lesson. If you have any errors, count them and write the number in the blank at the top of the page. Practice any missed or misspelled words on the next page. Sign your work and give it to your instructor. You are now ready for the next lesson.

PRACTICE

LESSON

44 Terminology Presentation

Listen to the Lab Tape provided by your instructor, and you will hear the words presented in this lesson. Read the words as they are said, noticing spelling and pronunciation. The recording will tell you when the presentation for this lesson is completed and will give you any further instructions. Do not go on to the next recorded lesson until you have completed Lesson 44 and feel that you know the words and word parts that have been presented.

••• ▸ *Start Audio*

sperm(a), sperm(i), sperm(o), spermat(o) a word element denoting a seed, usually the male generative element (semen)

WORD	WORD PART	DEFINITION	ANSWER
1. spermatorrhea (sper′mah-to-re′ah)	-rrhea	flow	1. ______
2. spermatopoietic (sper′mah-to-poi-et′ik)	-poiesis -ic	form, formation pertaining to	2. ______
3. spermatocyte (sper′mah-to-sit′)	-cyte	cell	3. ______
4. spermophlebectasia (sper′mo-fle′bek-ta′ze-ah)	phleb(o) -ectasia	vein dilatation, expansion	4. ______
5. spermatoschesis (sper′mah-tos′ke-sis)	-schesis	to check	5. ______
6. spermicide (sper′mi-sid)	-cide	death, killer	6. ______
7. spermatism (sper′mah-tizm)	-ism	condition	7. ______

ovari(o) a combining form denoting relationship to the ovary

WORD	WORD PART	DEFINITION	ANSWER
8. ovariocele (o-va′re-o-sel′)	-cele	tumor, swelling, hernia	8. ______

9. ovariocyesis (o-va're-o-si-e'sis)	-cyesis	pregnancy	9. ______
10. ovariosalpingectomy (o-va're-o-sal'pin-jek'to-me)	salping -ectomy	uterine tube excision, removal	10. ______
11. ovariorrhexis (o-va're-o-rek'sis)	-rrhexis	rupture	11. ______
12. ovariodysneuria (o-va're-o-dis-nu're-ah)	dys neur	abnormal, painful nerves	12. ______
13. ovariocentesis (o-va're-o-sen-te'sis)	-centesis	surgical puncture	13. ______
14. ovariopathy (o-va're-op'ah-the)	-pathy	disease	14. ______
15. ovariotubal (o-va're-o-tu'bal)	tub -al	tube of, pertaining to	15. ______

■ • • • *Stop Audio at Tone*

Study the 15 words and word parts for this lesson. Practice each word several times, checking your spelling and repeating the meaning to yourself. Listen to the recording and pronounce the words as many times as necessary. When you feel that you know the words and word parts well, you are ready to go on to the next step.

Use a sheet of paper to cover all columns except the Answer Column on the previous page. The words you have learned will be presented again on the recording. As each word is pronounced, write it in the space provided in the Answer Column.

• • • ▶ *Start Audio*

After stopping the tape player, check the words you have written against the words in the left-hand column. If any words are misspelled, practice writing them correctly. When you feel that you know and understand the words and word parts, go on to the Terminology Practice.

PRACTICE

Name ______________________ Date ______________ Errors ________

LESSON 44: TERMINOLOGY PRACTICE

Without looking at your previous work, write the word that is described by each definition.

sperm(a), sperm(o), sperm(i), spermat(o) and *ovari(o)*

DEFINITION	TERM
1. Rupture of an ovary	____________
2. Ovarian disease	____________
3. Promoting secretion of semen	____________
4. Removal of the ovary and oviduct	____________
5. Pertaining to the ovary and uterine tubes	____________
6. Dilatation or varicosity of the spermatic veins	____________
7. Pertaining to a condition in which semen is produced or discharged	____________
8. Hernial protrusion or tumor of an ovary	____________
9. Suppression of the secretion of semen	____________
10. An involuntary discharge of semen without orgasm	____________
11. Surgical puncture of an ovary	____________
12. An agent that is destructive to spermatozoa	____________
13. Neural pain in the ovary	____________
14. Ovarian pregnancy	____________
15. A sperm cell	____________

Check your answers against the word and definition lists on the first page of this lesson. If you have any errors, count them and write the number in the blank at the top of the page. Practice any missed or misspelled words on the next page. Sign your work and give it to your instructor. You are now ready for the next lesson.

PRACTICE

Name ______________________________ Date ____________________ Errors __________

LESSON 45 | TERMINOLOGY REVIEW FOR TEST 9

This is a review of the word parts you have learned in the preceding four lessons. Some of the medical terms listed below may be new, but they are made up of word parts that you have already learned. Read the words below as they are pronounced on the Lab Tape. As you listen, notice the familiar word parts which make them up.

• • • ▸ *Start Audio*

WORD	WORD PART	MEANING OF WORD PART
1. adenopathy	aden(o)	____________
(ad′e-nop′ah-the)	-pathy	____________
adenopathy	____________	
2. myxedema	myx(o)	____________
(mik′se-de′mah)	-edema	____________
myxedema	____________	
3. myxocyte	myx(o)	____________
(mik′so-sit)	-cyte	____________
myxocyte	____________	
4. galacturia	galact(o)	____________
(gal′ak-tu′re-ah)	-uria	____________
galacturia	____________	
5. adrenomegaly	adren(o)	____________
(ad-ren′o-meg′ah-le)	-megaly	____________
adrenomegaly	____________	
6. adrenalectomy	adrenal	____________
(ah-dre′nal-ek′to-me)	-ectomy	____________
adrenalectomy	____________	
7. pancreatalgia	pancreat(o)	____________
(pan′kre-ah-tal′je-ah)	-algia	____________
pancreatalgia	____________	
8. thyroglossal	thyr(o)	____________
(thi′ro-glos′al)	gloss(o)	____________
	-al	____________
thyroglossal	____________	

9. spermatoschesis (sper'mah-tos'ke-sis)
spermat(o) ____________
-schesis ____________
spermatoschesis ____________

10. ovariorrhexis (o-va're-o-rek'sis)
ovari(o) ____________
-rrhexis ____________
ovariorrhexis ____________

11. adenohypersthenia (ad'e-no-hi'per-sthe'ne-ah)
aden(o) ____________
hyper ____________
-sthenia ____________
adenohypersthenia ____________

12. galactophlysis (gal'ak-tof'li-sis)
galact(o) ____________
-phlysis ____________
galactophlysis ____________

13. adrenalinuria (ah-dren'ah-lin-u're-ah)
adrenalin ____________
-uria ____________
adrenalinuria ____________

14. pancreathelcosis (pan'kre-ath'el-ko'sis)
pancreat(o) ____________
helcosis ____________
pancreathelcosis ____________

15. spermophlebectasia (sper'mo-fle'bek-ta'ze-ah)
sperm(o) ____________
phleb(o) ____________
-ectasia ____________
spermophlebectasia ____________

■ • • • *Stop Audio at Tone*

On the lines provided, fill in the meanings of as many of the word parts as you can from memory. Then, use the previous lessons or a medical dictionary to look up any definitions you could not remember. Fill them in. On a separate piece of paper, practice writing the word parts and their meanings. Pay special attention to any which you had trouble remembering. Be sure to check your spelling.

When you have defined and reviewed all the word parts, write a definition for each whole word on the line provided. Check your definitions in the Glossary or a medical dictionary and make any needed corrections. Practice the words on a separate sheet of paper until you are sure that you know them. Then go on to the Extra Credit Review (if your instructor assigns it) or Test 9.

Name ______________________ Date ______________ Errors ________

LESSON 45 — **EXTRA CREDIT REVIEW**

This Extra Credit Review should be done at the discretion of your instructor. If you are instructed to complete this portion of the Review, turn it in to your instructor when you are finished.

PART A

Each phrase below defines one of the words you have just studied. Without looking at your previous work, fill in the word that matches each definition.

DEFINITION	TERM
1. Pancreatic pain	______________
2. The presence of adrenalin in the urine	______________
3. Any disease of the glands	______________
4. A vesicular eruption containing a milky fluid	______________
5. Pertaining to the thyroid and tongue	______________
6. Swelling due to mucus	______________
7. Suppression of the secretion of semen	______________
8. Excessive glandular activity	______________
9. Excision of the adrenal gland	______________
10. Enlargement of the adrenal gland	______________
11. Dilatation or varicosity of the spermatic veins	______________
12. Rupture of an ovary	______________
13. The discharge of milklike urine	______________
14. Ulceration of the pancreas	______________
15. A cell of mucous tissue	______________

PART B

Write the definition for the following terms to the right of the given term.

TERM	DEFINITION
16. adenocarcinoma	______________________
17. myxocystitis	______________________

18. thyrotoxicosis ____________________

19. ovariocyesis ____________________

20. adrenomegaly ____________________

21. adenoblast ____________________

22. pancreatopathy ____________________

23. ovariodysneuria ____________________

24. galactophoritis ____________________

25. adenemphraxis ____________________

26. pancreatitis ____________________

27. hypothyroidism ____________________

28. myxorrhea ____________________

29. spermatocyte ____________________

30. adrenokinetic ____________________

31. galactostasis ____________________

32. thyroptosis ____________________

33. adrenotoxin ____________________

34. pancreatectomy ____________________

35. galactacrasia ____________________

You may now go on to Test 9.

SECTION 10

Hemic and Lymphatic Systems

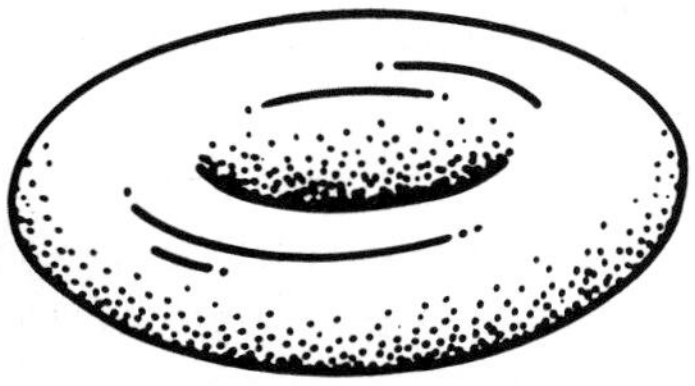

RED BLOOD CELLS
erythr(o) + cyte

BLOOD
hem(o)
hemat(o)
emia

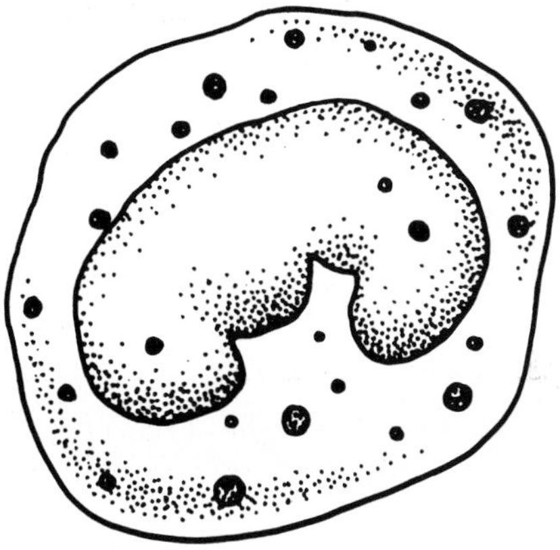

WHITE BLOOD CELLS
leuk(o) + cyte

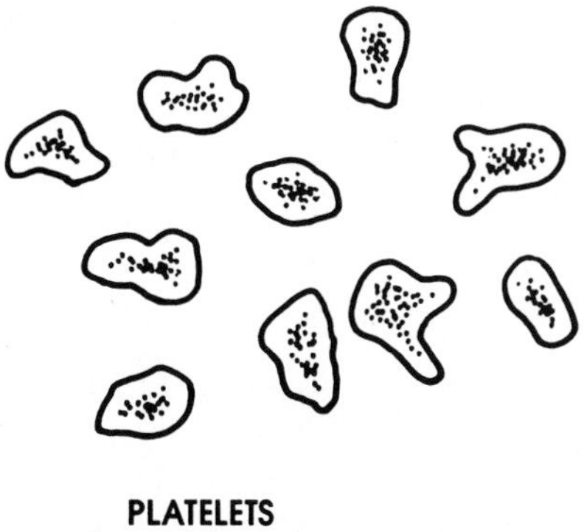

PLATELETS
thromb(o) + cyte

HEMIC AND LYMPHATIC SYSTEMS

Orientation

The hemic and lymphatic systems have to do with the blood and the lymph. Blood is made up of pale straw-colored fluid called plasma and various cells and cell parts (formed elements). The blood is about 55 percent plasma, which in turn is about 90 percent water. The remaining part of plasma contains protein. Some of these proteins are serum albumin, serum globulin, and fibrinogen.

The blood cells include erythrocytes (red blood cells), leukocytes (white blood cells), and platelets or thrombocytes. Erythrocytes contain the protein hemoglobin, which allows them to carry oxygen throughout the body. Iron is a very important part of red blood cells. Erythrocytes are formed in the red bone marrow.

Thrombocytes or platelets are important elements in the blood for coagulation or clotting. When a vessel is damaged or injured, the platelets form and release fibrin, a protein, which aids in clotting in this area.

There are several types of leukocytes, some of which consume foreign particles, such as bacteria and viruses, and others which produce antibodies. An increased amount of leukocytes in the bloodstream is often a sign of infection.

Lymph is a colorless liquid made up of fluid from the spaces between cells and various salts, sugar, water, and waste products. From all parts of the body, it enters special lymph vessels that transport the lymph to the heart area, where it is added to the blood. The lymph passes through nodular lymph glands, where harmful substances such as bacteria are filtered out. Lymph cells or lymphocytes are important in the body's immune system.

LESSON

46 Terminology Presentation

Listen to the Lab Tape provided by your instructor, and you will hear the words presented in this lesson. Read the words as they are said, noticing spelling and pronunciation. The recording will tell you when the presentation for this lesson is completed and will give you any further instructions. Do not go on to the next recorded lesson until you have completed Lesson 46 and feel that you know the words and word parts that have been presented.

• • • ▶ *Start Audio*

hem(o), hemat(o) a combining form denoting the blood

WORD	WORD PART	DEFINITION	ANSWER
1. hemarthrosis (hem′ar-thro′sis)	arthr(o) -osis	joint condition, process, increase, disease	1. ________
2. hemostat (he′mo-stat)	-stat	stop	2. ________
3. hematoscheocele (hem′ah-tos′ke-o-sel′)	scheo -cele	scrotum tumor, swelling, hernia	3. ________
4. hematocrit (he-mat′o-krit)	-crit	separate	4. ________
5. hemolysis (he-mol′i-sis)	-lysis	dissolve, break down	5. ________
6. hematemesis (hem′ah-tem-e-sis)	-emesis	vomit	6. ________
7. hemangioma (he-man′je-o′ma)	angi(o) -oma	vessels tumor	7. ________
8. hemoptysis (he-mop′ti-sis)	-ptysis	cough up, spit up	8. ________

splen(o) a combining form denoting the spleen

WORD	WORD PART	DEFINITION	ANSWER
9. splenophrenic (splen-o-fren'ik)	phren(o) -ic	diaphragm pertaining to	9. ______
10. splenoncus (sple-nong'kus)	-oncus	mass, bulk, tumor	10. ______
11. splenectomy (sple-nek'to-me)	-ectomy	excision, removal	11. ______
12. splenatrophy (splen-at'ro-fe)	a- -trophy	without, lack of nourishment	12. ______
13. splenohepatomegaly (sple'no-hep'ah-to-meg'ah-le)	hepat(o) -megaly	liver enlarge	13. ______
14. splenocele (sple'no-sel)	-cele	tumor, swelling, hernia	14. ______
15. splenorrhagia (sple'no-ra'je-ah)	-rrhagia	excessive flow, bleeding	15. ______

■ • • • *Stop Audio at Tone*

Study the 15 words and word parts for this lesson. Practice each word several times, checking your spelling and repeating the meaning to yourself. Listen to the recording and pronounce the words as many times as necessary. When you feel that you know the words and word parts well, you are ready to go on to the next step.

Use a sheet of paper to cover all columns except the Answer Column on the previous page. The words you have learned will be presented again on the recording. As each word is pronounced, write it in the space provided in the Answer Column.

• • • ▶ *Start Audio*

After stopping the tape player, check the words you have written against the words in the left-hand column. If any words are misspelled, practice writing them correctly. When you feel that you know and understand the words and word parts, go on to the Terminology Practice.

PRACTICE

______

______

______

Name ________________________________ Date ____________________ Errors __________

LESSON 46: TERMINOLOGY PRACTICE

Without looking at your previous work, write the word that is described by each definition.

hem(o), hemat(o) **and** ***splen(o)***

DEFINITION	TERM
1. Accumulation of blood in a joint cavity	____________
2. Bleeding or hemorrhage from the spleen	____________
3. Tumor of the spleen	____________
4. Spitting or coughing up blood	____________
5. An accumulation of blood in the scrotum	____________
6. An instrument or medicine for stopping bleeding	____________
7. Vomiting of blood	____________
8. A benign tumor composed of newly formed blood vessels	____________
9. The volume percentage of red cells to whole blood (separation of red cells for counting)	____________
10. Excision or removal of the spleen	____________
11. Pertaining to the spleen and diaphragm	____________
12. Atrophy or wasting of the spleen	____________
13. Enlargement of the spleen and liver	____________
14. Breaking down or destroying blood cells	____________
15. Herniation or swelling of the spleen	____________

Check your answers against the word and definition lists on the first page of this lesson. If you have any errors, count them and write the number in the blank at the top of the page. Practice any missed or misspelled words on the next page. Sign your work and give it to your instructor. You are now ready for the next lesson.

PRACTICE

LESSON 47

Terminology Presentation

Listen to the Lab Tape provided by your instructor, and you will hear the words presented in this lesson. Read the words as they are said, noticing spelling and pronunciation. The recording will tell you when the presentation for this lesson is completed and will give you any further instructions. Do not go on to the next recorded lesson until you have completed Lesson 47 and feel that you know the words and word parts that have been presented.

• • • ▶ *Start Audio*

angi(o) a word part indicating relationship to a vessel, usually a blood vessel

WORD	WORD PART	DEFINITION	ANSWER
1. angiectasis (an′je-ek′tah-sis)	-ectasis	dilatation, expansion	1. ________
2. angiostomy (an′je-os′to-me)	-stomy	connection, opening	2. ________
3. angiomyolipoma (an′je-o-mi′o-li-po′mah)	my(o) lip(o) -oma	muscle fat tumor	3. ________
4. angiospasm (an′je-o-spazm′)	-spasm	contraction	4. ________
5. angiogram (an′je-o-gram′)	-gram	something recorded	5. ________
6. angiomegaly (an′je-o-meg′ah-le)	megaly	enlargement	6. ________
7. angiostenosis (an′je-o-ste-no′sis)	-stenosis	narrowing	7. ________

emia a word element denoting relationship to the blood

WORD	WORD PART	DEFINITION	ANSWER
8. polycythemia (pol′e-si-the′me-ah)	poly cyt(e)	many, increase cell	8. ________

9. leukemia (loo-ke′me-ah)	leuk(o)	white	9. ________
10. lipemia (li-pe′me-ah)	lip(o)	fat	10. ________
11. hyperglycemia (hi′per-gli-se′me-ah)	hyper glyc(o)	above, over, abundant sugar	11. ________
12. anemia (ah-ne′me-ah)	an	without, lack of	12. ________
13. oligemia (ol′i-ge′me-ah)	olig(o)	few	13. ________
14. cyanemia (si′ah-ne′me-ah)	cyan(o)	blue	14. ________

■ • • • *Stop Audio at Tone*

Study the 14 words and word parts for this lesson. Practice each word several times, checking your spelling and repeating the meaning to yourself. Listen to the recording and pronounce the words as many times as necessary. When you feel that you know the words and word parts well, you are ready to go on to the next step.

Use a sheet of paper to cover all columns except the Answer Column on the previous page. The words you have learned will be presented again on the recording. As each word is pronounced, write it in the space provided in the Answer Column.

• • • ▶ *Start Audio*

After stopping the tape player, check the words you have written against the words in the left-hand column. If any words are misspelled, practice writing them correctly. When you feel that you know and understand the words and word parts, go on to the Terminology Practice.

PRACTICE

____

____

____

____

____

____

____

Name ______________________________ Date __________________ Errors __________

LESSON 47: TERMINOLOGY PRACTICE

Without looking at your previous work, write the word that is described by each definition.

angi(o) and *emia*

DEFINITION	TERM
1. Contraction of a blood vessel	______________
2. Deficiency in the volume of blood	______________
3. Enlarged blood vessels	______________
4. Abnormally high concentration of fat in the blood	______________
5. Dilatation of a blood vessel	______________
6. Increase in the number of red blood cells in the blood	______________
7. X-ray picture (roentgenogram) of a blood vessel	______________
8. Excessive number of white blood cells	______________
9. Tumor of blood vessels, muscle, and fat	______________
10. Bluishness of the blood	______________
11. Narrowing of the lumen (inside) of a blood vessel	______________
12. Excessive sugar in the blood	______________
13. Reduction in the number of red blood cells in the blood	______________
14. Making an opening into the blood vessel	______________

Check your answers against the word and definition lists on the first page of this lesson. If you have any errors, count them and write the number in the blank at the top of the page. Practice any missed or misspelled words on the next page. Sign your work and give it to your instructor. You are now ready for the next lesson.

PRACTICE

LESSON

48 Terminology Presentation

Listen to the Lab Tape provided by your instructor, and you will hear the words presented in this lesson. Read the words as they are said, noticing spelling and pronunciation. The recording will tell you when the presentation for this lesson is completed and will give you any further instructions. Do not go on to the next recorded lesson until you have completed Lesson 48 and feel that you know the words and word parts that have been presented.

• • • ▶ *Start Audio*

lymph(o) a combining form indicating lymph or the lymphatic glands or vessels

WORD	WORD PART	DEFINITION	ANSWER
1. lymphadenitis (lim-fad′e-ni′tis)	aden(o) -itis	gland inflammation	1. ________
2. lymphopathy (lim-fop′ah-the)	-pathy	disease	2. ________
3. lymphangioma (lim-fan′je-o′mah)	angi(o) -oma	vessel tumor	3. ________
4. lymphocyte (lim′fo-sit)	-cyte	cell	4. ________
5. lymphocytopenia (lim′fo-si′to-pe′ne-ah)	cyt(o) -penia	cell decrease	5. ________
6. lymphopoiesis (lim′fo-poi-e′sis)	-poiesis	form, formation	6. ________
7. lymphedema (lim′fe-de′mah)	-edema	swelling	7. ________
8. lymphostasis (lim-fos′tah-sis)	-stasis	stop	8. ________

phil(ia) a word ending denoting love or attraction to

WORD	WORD PART	DEFINITION	ANSWER
9. polychromatophilia (pol′e-kro′mah-to-fil′e-ah)	poly	many	9. ________
	chromat(o)	color	
10. eosinophil (e′o-sin′o-fil)	eosin(o)	rose colored	10. ________
11. hemophilia (he′mo-fil′e-ah)	hem(o)	blood	11. ________
12. basophil (ba′so-fil)	bas(o)	basic	12. ________
13. pedophilia (pe′do-fil′e-ah)	ped(o)	children	13. ________
14. neutrophil (nu′tro-fil)	neutr(o)	neither	14. ________
15. hydrophilic (hi′dro-fil′ik)	hydr(o)	water	15. ________

■ • • • *Stop Audio at Tone*

Study the 15 words and word parts for this lesson. Practice each word several times, checking your spelling and repeating the meaning to yourself. Listen to the recording and pronounce the words as many times as necessary. When you feel that you know the words and word parts well, you are ready to go on to the next step.

Use a sheet of paper to cover all columns except the Answer Column on the previous page. The words you have learned will be presented again on the recording. As each word is pronounced, write it in the space provided in the Answer Column.

• • • ▶ *Start Audio*

After stopping the tape player, check the words you have written against the words in the left-hand column. If any words are misspelled, practice writing them correctly. When you feel that you know and understand the words and word parts, go on to the Terminology Practice.

PRACTICE

____

____

____

Name ______________________ Date ______________ Errors ________

LESSON 48: TERMINOLOGY PRACTICE

Without looking at your previous work, write the word that is described by each definition.

lymph(o) and *phil(ia)*

DEFINITION	TERM
1. Swelling of subcutaneous tissue due to excessive lymph fluid	______________
2. Making or developing lymph	______________
3. The quality of being stainable with various stains or colors	______________
4. A cell or structure staining readily with basic dyes	______________
5. A disease in which the blood clots slowly (bleeder's disease)	______________
6. Inflammation of the lymph gland	______________
7. Reduction in the number of lymphocytes in the blood	______________
8. Attracted or stainable with a rose-colored dye or stain	______________
9. Stoppage of lymph flow	______________
10. A tumor rich in blood vessels	______________
11. Any disease of the lymphatic system	______________
12. Readily stainable with a neutral stain	______________
13. Attracts or absorbs water	______________
14. A morbid sexual perversion toward children	______________
15. A white cell which is formed in the lymph glands	______________

Check your answers against the word and definition lists on the first page of this lesson. If you have any errors, count them and write the number in the blank at the top of the page. Practice any missed or misspelled words in the space provided. Sign your work and give it to your instructor. You are now ready for the next lesson.

PRACTICE

LESSON

49 Terminology Presentation

Listen to the Lab Tape provided by your instructor, and you will hear the words presented in this lesson. Read the words as they are said, noticing spelling and pronunciation. The recording will tell you when the presentation for this lesson is completed and will give you any further instructions. Do not go on to the next recorded lesson until you have completed Lesson 49 and feel that you know the words and word parts that have been presented.

• • • ▸ *Start Audio*

erythr(o) a word element denoting red or red blood cells

WORD	WORD PART	DEFINITION	ANSWER
1. erythrocyte (e-rith′ro-sit)	-cyte	cell	1. ________
2. erythropenia (e-rith′ro-pe′ne-ah)	-penia	decrease	2. ________
3. erythropoiesis (e-rith′ro-poi-e′sis)	-poiesis	form, formation	3. ________
4. erythroclasis (er′e-throk′lah-sis)	-clasis	break, fracture	4. ________
5. erythrocytosis (e-rith′ro-si-to′sis)	-cytosis	increase in cells	5. ________
6. erythrodontia (e-rith′ro-don′she-ah)	odontia	teeth, tooth	6. ________
7. erythroderma (e-rith′ro-der′mah)	derm(a)	skin	7. ________
8. erythroblast (e-rith′ro-blast)	-blast	immature cell	8. ________

cyt(o) a combining form denoting relationship to a cell

WORD	WORD PART	DEFINITION	ANSWER
9. cytobiology (si′to-bi-ol′o-je)	bi(o) -logy	life, living study of, science of	9. ________

10. cytotoxicity (si′to-tok-sis′i-te)	-toxicity	poison	**10.** ________
11. cytodiagnosis (si′to-di′ag-no′sis)	dia -gnosis	through knowledge	**11.** ________
12. cytometaplasia (si′to-met′ah-pla′ze-ah)	meta -plasia	change formation	**12.** ________
13. cytomorphology (si′to-mor-fol′o-je)	morph(o) -logy	shape, form study of, science of	**13.** ________
14. cytolysis (si-tol′i-sis)	-lysis	dissolve, break	**14.** ________
15. cytoma (si-to′mah)	-oma	tumor	**15.** ________

■ • • • *Stop Audio at Tone*

Study the 15 words and word parts for this lesson. Practice each word several times, checking your spelling and repeating the meaning to yourself. Listen to the recording and pronounce the words as many times as necessary. When you feel that you know the words and word parts well, you are ready to go on to the next step.

Use a sheet of paper to cover all columns except the Answer Column on the previous page. The words you have learned will be presented again on the recording. As each word is pronounced, write it in the space provided in the Answer Column.

• • • ▶ *Start Audio*

After stopping the tape player, check the words you have written against the words in the left-hand column. If any words are misspelled, practice writing them correctly. When you feel that you know and understand the words and word parts, go on to the Terminology Practice.

PRACTICE

Name ______________________ Date ______________ Errors ________

LESSON 49: TERMINOLOGY PRACTICE

Without looking at your previous work, write the word that is described by each definition.

erythr(o) and *cyt(o)*

DEFINITION	TERM
1. Breaking up or splitting up of red cells	______________
2. Being poisonous or toxic to cells	______________
3. The biology of cells	______________
4. Abnormal redness of the skin over wide areas of the body	______________
5. Study of the shape of cells	______________
6. A red blood cell	______________
7. Reddish brown pigmentation of the teeth	______________
8. An immature red cell	______________
9. Diagnosis of disease by examination of cells	______________
10. Destruction or dissolution of cells	______________
11. Forming or manufacturing of red blood cells	______________
12. A cell tumor	______________
13. Deficiency in the number of red blood cells	______________
14. An increase in red blood cells	______________
15. Change in the form or function of a cell	______________

Check your answers against the word and definition lists on the first page of this lesson. If you have any errors, count them and write the number in the blank at the top of the page. Practice any missed or misspelled words on the next page. Sign your work and give it to your instructor. You are now ready for the next lesson.

PRACTICE

Name ______________________ Date ______________ Errors __________

LESSON 50 — TERMINOLOGY REVIEW FOR TEST 10

This is a review of the word parts you have learned in the preceding four lessons. Some of the medical terms listed below may be new, but they are made up of word parts that you have already learned.

Unlike the review for Test 9, the words are not written out for you. As each word is pronounced on the Lab Tape, write it in the appropriate numbered blank on the left.

• • • ▶ *Start Audio*

WORD	WORD PART	MEANING OF WORD PART
1. ____________	________	________________
	________	________________
	________	________________
2. ____________	________	________________
	________	________________
	________	________________
3. ____________	________	________________
	________	________________
	________	________________
4. ____________	________	________________
	________	________________
	________	________________
5. ____________	________	________________
	________	________________
	________	________________
6. ____________	________	________________
	________	________________
	________	________________
7. ____________	________	________________
	________	________________
	________	________________
8. ____________	________	________________
	________	________________
	________	________________

9. ______________________ ______________ ________________________________
______________ ________________________________
______________ ________________________________

10. ______________________ ______________ ________________________________
______________ ________________________________
______________ ________________________________

11. ______________________ ______________ ________________________________
______________ ________________________________
______________ ________________________________

12. ______________________ ______________ ________________________________
______________ ________________________________
______________ ________________________________

13. ______________________ ______________ ________________________________
______________ ________________________________
______________ ________________________________

14. ______________________ ______________ ________________________________
______________ ________________________________
______________ ________________________________

15. ______________________ ______________ ________________________________
______________ ________________________________
______________ ________________________________

■ • • • *Stop Audio at Tone*

After all 15 words have been written, write the word parts for each one and fill in the meanings of the parts. Use the Glossary or a medical dictionary to check your spellings and definitions. Practice the words on a separate sheet of paper, paying particular attention to any you missed or misspelled.

When you feel you know the words and word parts well, sign your work, indicate the number of errors, and turn your work in to your instructor.

You are now ready for the Extra Credit Review (if your instructor assigns it) or Test 10.

Name ______________________ Date ______________ Errors ________

LESSON 50 | EXTRA CREDIT REVIEW

This Extra Credit Review should be done at the discretion of your instructor. If you are instructed to complete this portion of the Review, turn it in to your instructor when you are finished.

PART A

Write the proper term for the following 20 definitions to the right of the given definition.

DEFINITION	TERM
1. Vomiting of blood	______________
2. Change in the form or function of cells	______________
3. Abnormal redness of the skin over wide areas of the body	______________
4. Enlargement of the spleen and liver	______________
5. An instrument or medicine for stopping bleeding	______________
6. X-ray picture (roentgenogram) of a blood vessel	______________
7. Reduction in the number of lymphocytes in the blood	______________
8. Increase in the number of red blood cells in the blood	______________
9. An accumulation of blood in the scrotum	______________
10. Removal of the spleen	______________
11. Tumor of blood vessels, muscle, and fat	______________
12. The biology of cells	______________
13. A cell or structure readily stainable with basic dyes	______________
14. Being poisonous or toxic to cells	______________
15. Breaking up or splitting of red blood cells	______________
16. Attracted to or stainable with a rose-colored dye or stain	______________
17. Bluishness of the blood	______________

18. A cell tumor ______________________

19. An immature red cell ______________________

20. Inflammation of the lymph gland ______________________

PART B

Match the following terms with the definitions given. Place the correct letter of the term to the left of the definition.

DEFINITION	TERM
______ 21. Herniation or swelling of the spleen	a. angiostenosis
______ 22. Reduction in the number of red blood cells in the blood	b. lymphocyte
______ 23. Increase in the number of red blood cells in the blood	c. hemoptysis
______ 24. Spitting or coughing up blood	d. polycythemia
______ 25. Bleeding or hemorrhage from the spleen	e. hemophilia
______ 26. Narrowing of the lumen of a blood vessel	f. splenocele
______ 27. Study of the shape of cells	g. erythropenia
______ 28. Deficiency in the number of red blood cells	h. anemia
______ 29. A white cell which is formed in the lymph glands	i. splenorrhagia
______ 30. A disease in which the blood clots slowly	j. cytomorphology

You may now go on to Test 10.

SECTION

11 Numbers, Amounts, Colors and Positions

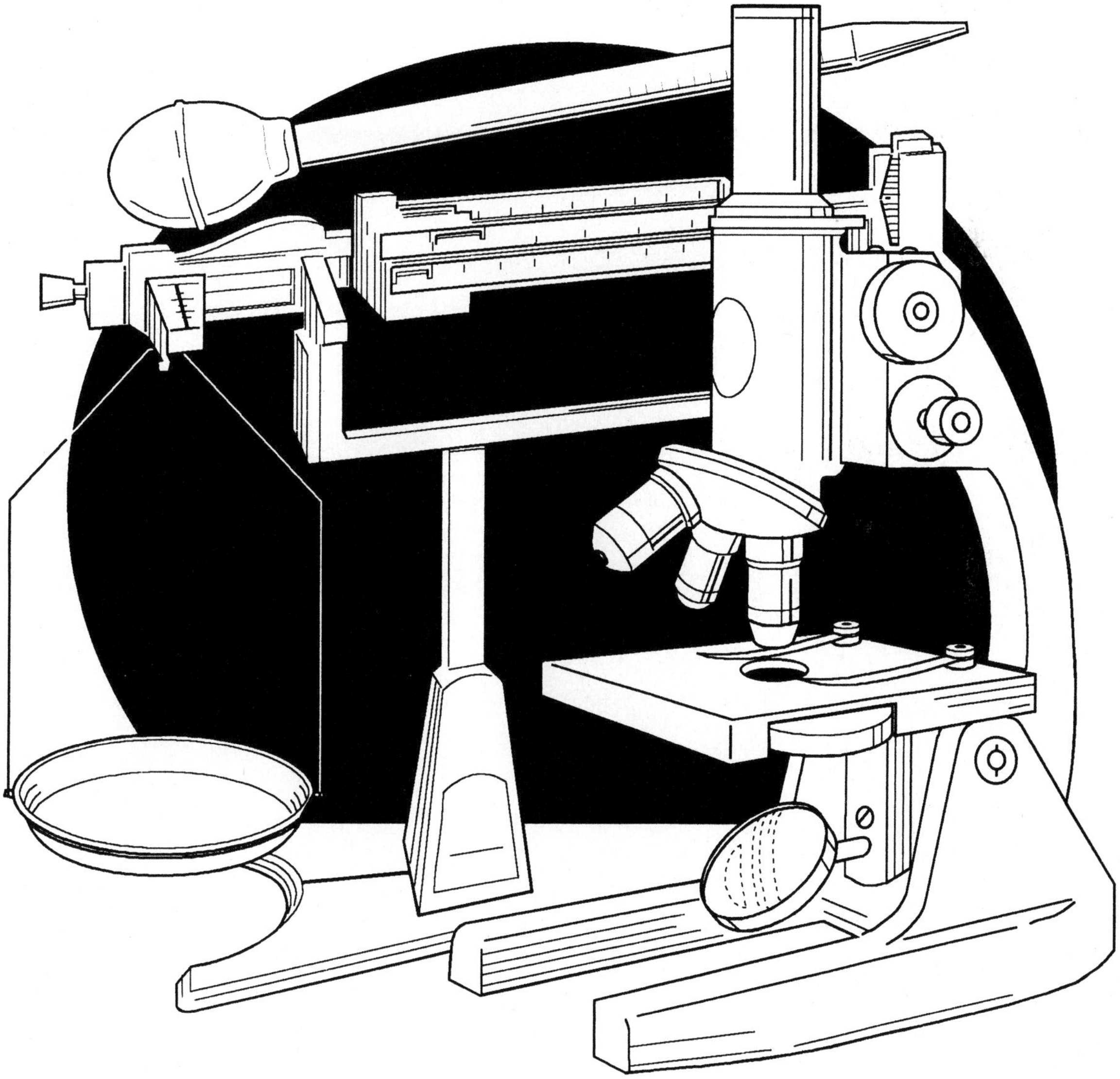

NUMBERS, AMOUNTS, COLORS, AND POSITIONS

Orientation

This section involves numbers, amounts, colors, and positions. Numbers are quite important for anyone working in the medical field, since they are commonly used in lab reports and many physicians' reports to denote weights and measurements.

Amounts and colors are also used in many types of medical reports. Such terms as rubella indicate a given disease. Many disease symptoms use colors to identify them (purpura). The use of the proper word part or parts denoting color are also widely used in identifying laboratory findings such as eosinophilia.

Positions such as supra, infra, etc., are commonly used in anatomical descriptions. Many physicians' reports use these positions to indicate the site of a symptom or injury to the body.

LESSON 51

Terminology Presentation

Numbers

This lesson presents 14 different words that indicate numbers. Listen to the Lab Tape provided by your instructor, and you will hear the words presented in this lesson. Read the words as they are said, noticing spelling and pronunciation. The recording will tell you when the presentation for this lesson is completed and will give you any further instructions. Do not go on to the next recorded lesson until you have completed Lesson 51 and feel that you know the words and word parts that have been presented.

• • • ▸ ***Start Audio***

WORD	WORD PART	DEFINITION	ANSWER
1. octipara (ok-tip'ah-rah)	oct(o) -para	eight (8) bring forth, produce	1. ________
2. centimeter (sen'ti-me'ter)	centi- -meter	100 or 1/100 measure (1 meter = 39.37 inches)	2. ________
3. hectogram (hek'to-gram)	hect(o)- -gram	100 weight (1 gram = 0.035 oz.)	3. ________
4. kilounit (kil'o-u'nit)	kilo- -unit	1000 unit	4. ________
5. quinquecuspid (kwin'kwe-kus'pid)	quinqu(e) cuspid	five (5) point	5. ________
6. millivolt (mil'i-volt)	milli- -volt	1/1000 volt (electric force)	6. ________
7. decagram (dek'ah-gram)	deca- -gram	10 weight (1 gram = 0.035 oz.)	7. ________
8. demilune (dem'e-lun)	demi- -lune	half (1/2) moon, crescent	8. ________
9. deciliter (des'i-le'ter)	deci- -liter	1/10 measure (1 liter = 1.0567 quarts)	9. ________
10. tetradactyly (tet'rah-dak'ti-le)	tetra- -dactyl(o)	four (4) finger, toe, digit	10. ________

11. pentachromic (pen′tah-kro′mik)	penta- chrom -ic	five (5) color pertaining to	**11.** ________________
12. triorchidism (tri-or′ki-dizm)	tri- orchid(o) -ism	three (3) testes, testicle condition	**12.** ________________
13. hemianesthesia (hem′e-an′es-the′ze-ah)	hemi- an- -esthesia	half (1/2) without, lack of perception, sense	**13.** ________________
14. quadruped (kwod′roo-ped)	quadr(u)- ped(o)	four (4) foot, feet	**14.** ________________

■ • • • *Stop Audio at Tone*

Study the 14 words and word parts for this lesson. Practice each word several times, checking your spelling and repeating the meaning to yourself. Listen to the recording and pronounce the words as many times as necessary. When you feel that you know the words and word parts well, you are ready to go on to the next step.

Use a sheet of paper to cover all columns except the Answer Column on the previous page. The words you have learned will be presented again on the recording. As each word is pronounced, write it in the space provided in the Answer Column.

• • • ▶ *Start Audio*

After stopping the tape player, check the words you have written against the words in the left-hand column. If any words are misspelled, practice writing them correctly. When you feel that you know and understand the words and word parts, go on to the Terminology Practice.

PRACTICE

Name ______________________ Date ______________ Errors ________

LESSON 51: TERMINOLOGY PRACTICE

Numbers

Without looking at your previous work, write the word that is described by each definition.

DEFINITION	TERM
1. A tooth having five points or cusps	______________
2. A unit of mass being 100 grams	______________
3. The condition of having four digits on the hands or feet	______________
4. One-tenth of a liter	______________
5. Half moon or crescent shaped	______________
6. The condition of having three testes	______________
7. A unit of the metric system being one-hundredth part of a meter	______________
8. 1/1000 of a volt	______________
9. A woman who has had eight pregnancies	______________
10. A quantity equaling 1000 units	______________
11. Condition denoting anesthesia (lack of feeling) on one side of the body	______________
12. Ten grams	______________
13. Pertaining to or exhibiting five colors	______________
14. Four footed, such as many animals	______________

Check your answers against the word and definition lists on the first page of this lesson. If you have any errors, count them and write the number in the blank at the top of the page. Practice any missed or misspelled words on the next page. Sign your work and give it to your instructor. You are now ready for the next lesson.

PRACTICE

LESSON

52

Terminology Presentation

Amounts and Positions, Part 1

This lesson presents 14 different words that indicate amounts and positions. Listen to the Lab Tape provided by your instructor, and you will hear the words presented in this lesson. Read the words as they are said, noticing spelling and pronunciation. The recording will tell you when the presentation for this lesson is completed and will give you any further instructions. Do not go on to the next recorded lesson until you have completed Lesson 52 and feel that you know the words and word parts that have been presented.

• • • ▸ *Start Audio*

WORD	WORD PART	DEFINITION	ANSWER
1. anterosuperior (an′ter-o-su-per′e-or)	anter(o)- super(ior)	before above	1. ________
2. apobiosis (ap′o-bi-o′sis)	ap(o)- bi(o) -osis	separation, deviation life condition, process, increase, disease	2. ________
3. anastomosis (ah-nas′to-mo′sis)	ana- -stoma -osis	up mouth, opening condition, process, increase, disease	3. ________
4. cataphasia (kat′ah-fa′ze-ah)	cata- -phasia	down speech	4. ________
5. antiemetic (an′ti-e-met′ik)	anti- emetic	against vomit	5. ________
6. inframammary (in′frah-mam′ah-re)	infra- mammary	below, beneath breast	6. ________
7. semicoma (sem′e-ko′mah)	semi- coma	half (1/2) stupor, unconscious	7. ________
8. contraindication (kon′trah-in′di-ka′shun)	contr(a) indicati(o)	against indicate, point to	8. ________
9. sublingual (sub-ling′gwal)	sub- lingu(a) -al	under tongue of, pertaining to	9. ________

10. supratympanic (soo'prah-tim-pan'ik)	supra- tympan(o) -ic	above tympanum, eardrum pertaining to	10. ________________
11. ambilateral (am'bi-lat'er-al)	ambi- -lateral	both side	11. ________________
12. tertian (ter'shun)	ter(ti)- -an	three (3) pertaining to	12. ________________
13. ultrasonic (ul'trah-son'ik)	ultra- son(o) -ic	above, excess sound pertaining to	13. ________________
14. unilateral (u'ni-lat'er-al)	uni- -lateral	one side	14. ________________

■ • • • *Stop Audio at Tone*

Study the 14 words and word parts for this lesson. Practice each word several times, checking your spelling and repeating the meaning to yourself. Listen to the recording and pronounce the words as many times as necessary. When you feel that you know the words and word parts well, you are ready to go on to the next step.

Use a sheet of paper to cover all columns except the Answer Column on the previous page. The words you have learned will be presented again on the recording. As each word is pronounced, write it in the space provided in the Answer Column.

• • • ▶ *Start Audio*

After stopping the tape player, check the words you have written against the words in the left-hand column. If any words are misspelled, practice writing them correctly. When you feel that you know and understand the words and word parts, go on to the Terminology Practice.

PRACTICE

____

____

____

____

____

____

____

____

Name ______________________ Date ______________ Errors ________

LESSON 52: TERMINOLOGY PRACTICE

Amounts and Positions, Part 1

Without looking at your previous work, write the word that is described by each definition.

DEFINITION	TERM
1. Not living—physiological death	______________
2. Situated beneath the tongue	______________
3. Recurring every third day	______________
4. Situated in front and above something	______________
5. Pertaining to both the right and left side	______________
6. A speech disorder in which the same word or phrase is constantly repeated	______________
7. An opening or connection between two vessels or organs	______________
8. Having a frequency above sound	______________
9. Any condition which renders a certain treatment undesirable or not indicated	______________
10. A stupor from which the patient may be aroused	______________
11. Situated above the tympanum	______________
12. An agent that prevents or alleviates nausea and vomiting	______________
13. Situated beneath the breast	______________
14. Pertaining to or affecting only one side	______________

Check your answers against the word and definition lists on the first page of this lesson. If you have any errors, count them and write the number in the blank at the top of the page. Practice any missed or misspelled words on the next page. Sign your work and give it to your instructor. You are now ready for the next lesson.

PRACTICE

LESSON

53 Terminology Presentation

Amounts and Positions, Part 2

This lesson presents 14 different words that indicate amounts and positions. Listen to the Lab Tape provided by your instructor, and you will hear the words presented in this lesson. Read the words as they are said, noticing spelling and pronunciation. The recording will tell you when the presentation for this lesson is completed and will give you any further instructions. Do not go on to the next recorded lesson until you have completed Lesson 53 and feel that you know the words and word parts that have been presented.

• • • ▸ *Start Audio*

WORD	WORD PART	DEFINITION	ANSWER
1. diplophonia (dip′lo-fo′ne-ah)	dipl(o)- -phonia	double voice, sound	1. ______________
2. ectoderm (ek′to-derm)	ect(o) derm	outside skin	2. ______________
3. intercostal (in′ter-kos′tal)	inter- cost(o)- -al	between rib of, pertaining to	3. ______________
4. intrabuccal (in′trah-buk′al)	intra- bucc(o)- -al	within cheek, mouth of, pertaining to	4. ______________
5. epiotic (ep′e-ot′ik)	epi- otic	above, upon pertaining to the ear	5. ______________
6. monochromatic (mon′o-kro-mat′ik)	mon(o)- chromat(o)- -ic	one (1) color pertaining to	6. ______________
7. panhysterectomy (pan′his-ter-ek′to-me)	pan- hyster(o)-	all uterus	7. ______________
8. pericardium (per′i-kar′de-um)	peri- cardi(o)	around heart	8. ______________
9. pleocytosis (ple′o-si-to′sis)	ple(o)- cytosis	more, many cellular content	9. ______________
10. polyphagia (pol′e-fa′je-ah)	poly- -phagia	many to eat	10. ______________

11. protoplasia (pro-to-pla'se-ah)	prot(o)- -plasia	first formation	**11.** ____________
12. postmortem (post-mor'tem)	post- -mortem	after death	**12.** ____________
13. retractor (re-trak'tor)	re- -tract(or)	back to draw or pull, to hold	**13.** ____________
14. retroflexed (ret'ro-flekst)	retr(o)- -flexed	backward bent	**14.** ____________

■ • • • *Stop Audio at Tone*

Study the 14 words and word parts for this lesson. Practice each word several times, checking your spelling and repeating the meaning to yourself. Listen to the recording and pronounce the words as many times as necessary. When you feel that you know the words and word parts well, you are ready to go on to the next step.

Use a sheet of paper to cover all columns except the Answer Column on the previous page. The words you have learned will be presented again on the recording. As each word is pronounced, write it in the space provided in the Answer Column.

• • • ▶ *Start Audio*

After stopping the tape player, check the words you have written against the words in the left-hand column. If any words are misspelled, practice writing them correctly. When you feel that you know and understand the words and word parts, go on to the Terminology Practice.

PRACTICE

Name ______________________ Date ______________ Errors ________

LESSON 53: TERMINOLOGY PRACTICE

Amounts and Positions, Part 2

Without looking at your previous work, write the word that is described by each definition.

DEFINITION	TERM
1. The outermost of the layers of skin	________________
2. The production of double vocal sounds	________________
3. Presence of a greater number of cells than normal	________________
4. The fibroserous sac surrounding the heart	________________
5. Situated between the ribs	________________
6. The primary formation of tissue	________________
7. Occurring or performed after death	________________
8. Bent backwards	________________
9. Within the cheek or mouth	________________
10. An instrument to draw back and hold the edges of a wound	________________
11. Having only one color	________________
12. Situated above or upon the ear	________________
13. Total removal of the uterus and cervix (total hysterectomy)	________________
14. Excessive or overeating (bulimia)	________________

Check your answers against the word and definition lists on the first page of this lesson. If you have any errors, count them and write the number in the blank at the top of the page. Practice any missed or misspelled words on the next page. Sign your work and give it to your instructor. You are now ready for the next lesson.

PRACTICE

LESSON

54

Terminology Presentation

Colors and Positions

This lesson presents 12 different words that indicate colors and positions. Listen to the Lab Tape provided by your instructor, and you will hear the words presented in this lesson. Read the words as they are said, noticing spelling and pronunciation. The recording will tell you when the presentation for this lesson is completed and will give you any further instructions. Do not go on to the next recorded lesson until you have completed Lesson 54 and feel that you know the words and word parts that have been presented.

• • • ▸ *Start Audio*

	WORD	WORD PART	DEFINITION	ANSWER
1.	aboral (ab-o′ral)	ab- oral	away from mouth	1. ______
2.	adduct (ah-dukt′)	ad- -duct(o)	toward to draw	2. ______
3.	amaurosis (am′aw-ro′sis)	amaur(o) -osis	darkness condition, process, increase, disease	3. ______
4.	biceps (bi′seps)	bi- ceps	two, double head	4. ______
5.	dorsal (dor′sal)	dors(o) -al	back (of the body) of, pertaining to	5. ______
6.	dehydrate (de-hi′drat)	de- hydr(o)	from, not, down water	6. ______
7.	chlorophyll (klo′ro-fil)	chlor(o)- -phyll(o)	green leaf	7. ______
8.	cirrhosis (sir-ro′sis)	cirrh(o) -osis	yellow condition, process, increase, disease	8. ______
9.	glaucoma (glaw-ko′mah)	glauc(o) -oma	gray-green tumor (swelling)	9. ______
10.	purpuriferous (pur′pu-rif′er-us)	purpur- -iferous	purple bear, produce	10. ______

11. rubeosis (roo′be-o′sis)	rub(e) -osis	red condition, process, increase, disease	**11.** ________________
12. xanthochromic (zan′tho-kro′mik)	xanth(o)- chrom(o)- -ic	yellow color pertaining to	**12.** ________________

■ • • • *Stop Audio at Tone*

Study the 12 words and word parts for this lesson. Practice each word several times, checking your spelling and repeating the meaning to yourself. Listen to the recording and pronounce the words as many times as necessary. When you feel that you know the words and word parts well, you are ready to go on to the next step.

Use a sheet of paper to cover all columns except the Answer Column on the previous page. The words you have learned will be presented again on the recording. As each word is pronounced, write it in the space provided in the Answer Column.

• • • ▶ *Start Audio*

After stopping the tape player, check the words you have written against the words in the left-hand column. If any words are misspelled, practice writing them correctly. When you feel that you know and understand the words and word parts, go on to the Terminology Practice.

PRACTICE

Name ______________________ Date ______________ Errors ________

LESSON 54: TERMINOLOGY PRACTICE

Colors and Positions

Without looking at your previous work, write the word that is described by each definition.

DEFINITION	TERM
1. The green coloring matter of plants	______________
2. Blindness, inability to see	______________
3. A liver disorder in which a primary symptom is jaundice (yellow skin)	______________
4. Opacity of the crystalline lens of the eye in which the eye shows a gray-green color	______________
5. Redness of an area	______________
6. Denoting a yellow discoloration of the spinal fluid	______________
7. To draw toward	______________
8. Situated away from or remote from the mouth	______________
9. Producing a purple pigment	______________
10. To remove water from a substance, such as the body	______________
11. Pertaining to the back of the body	______________
12. A muscle having two heads	______________

Check your answers against the word and definition lists on the first page of this lesson. If you have any errors, count them and write the number in the blank at the top of the page. Practice any missed or misspelled words on the next page. Sign your work and give it to your instructor. You are now ready for the next lesson.

PRACTICE

Name ______________________ Date ______________ Errors ________

LESSON 55 | TERMINOLOGY REVIEW FOR TEST 11

This is a review of the word parts you have learned in the preceding four lessons. Some of the medical terms listed below may be new, but they are made up of word parts that you have already learned. Read the words below as they are pronounced on the Lab Tape. As you listen, notice the familiar word parts which make them up.

• • • ▸ *Start Audio*

WORD	WORD PART	MEANING OF WORD PART
1. hemianesthesia	hemi-	______________
(hem′e-an′es-the′ze-ah)	an-	______________
	-esthesia	______________
hemianesthesia	______________	______________
2. tertian	ter(ti)-	______________
(ter′shun)	-an	______________
tertian	______________	______________
3. protoplasia	prot(o)	______________
(pro-to-pla′ze-ah)	-plasia	______________
protoplasia	______________	______________
4. biceps	bi-	______________
(bi′seps)	ceps	______________
biceps	______________	______________
5. rubeosis	rub(e)	______________
(roo′be-o′sis)	-osis	______________
rubeosis	______________	______________
6. polyphagia	poly-	______________
(pol′e-fa′je-ah)	-phagia	______________
polyphagia	______________	______________
7. aboral	ab-	______________
(ab-o′ral)	oral	______________
aboral	______________	______________
8. infracostal	infra-	______________
(in′frah-kos′tal)	cost(o)	______________
	-al	______________
infracostal	______________	______________

9. centimeter (sen′ti-me′ter) — centi- ______ ; -meter ______
centimeter ______

10. anastomosis (ah-nas′to-mo′sis) — ana- ______ ; -stoma ______ ; -osis ______
anastomosis ______

11. antiemetic (an′ti-e-met′ik) — anti- ______ ; -emetic ______
antiemetic ______

12. postmortem (post-mor′tem) — post- ______ ; -mortem ______
postmortem ______

13. chlorophyll (klo′ro-fil) — chlor(o)- ______ ; -phyll(o) ______
chlorophyll ______

14. xanthochromic (zan′tho-kro′mik) — xanth(o)- ______ ; chrom(o) ______ ; -ic ______
xanthochromic ______

15. pentachromic (pen′tah-kro′mik) — penta- ______ ; chrom(o)- ______ ; -ic ______
pentachromic ______

■ • • • *Stop Audio at Tone*

On the lines provided, fill in the meanings of as many of the word parts as you can from memory. Then, use the previous lessons or a medical dictionary to look up any definitions you could not remember. Fill them in. On a separate piece of paper, practice writing the word parts and their meanings. Pay special attention to any which you had trouble remembering. Be sure to check your spelling.

When you have defined and reviewed all the word parts, write a definition for each whole word on the line provided. Check your definitions in the Glossary or a medical dictionary and make any needed corrections. Practice the words on a separate sheet of paper until you are sure that you know them. Then go on to the Extra Credit Review (if your instructor assigns it) or Test 11.

Name ________________________ Date ________________ Errors ________

LESSON 55 EXTRA CREDIT REVIEW

This Extra Credit Review should be done at the discretion of your instructor. If you are instructed to complete this portion of the Review, turn it in to your instructor when you are finished.

PART A

Each phrase below defines one of the words you have just studied. Without looking at your previous work, fill in the word that matches each definition.

DEFINITION	TERM
1. An agent that prevents or alleviates nausea and vomiting	________________
2. Redness of an area	________________
3. Situated below a rib	________________
4. Denoting a yellow discoloration of the spinal fluid	________________
5. Condition denoting anesthesia (lack of feeling) on one side of the body	________________
6. An opening or connection between two vessels or organs	________________
7. Overeating	________________
8. The green coloring matter of plants	________________
9. Recurring every third day	________________
10. The primary formation of tissue	________________
11. Pertaining to or exhibiting five colors	________________
12. A muscle having two heads	________________
13. A unit of the metric system being 1/100 of a meter	________________
14. Occurring or performed after death	________________
15. Situated away from or remote from the mouth	________________

PART B

Match the following terms with the definitions given. Place the correct letter of the term to the left of the definition.

DEFINITION		TERM
______ 16.	Producing a purple pigment	a. intrabuccal
______ 17.	The primary formation of tissue	b. epiotic
______ 18.	A tooth having five points or cusps	c. millivolt
______ 19.	Situated above or upon the ear	d. purpuriferous
______ 20.	Within the cheek or mouth	e. octipara
______ 21.	Situated beneath the breast	f. cirrhosis
______ 22.	A woman who has had eight pregnancies	g. protoplasia
______ 23.	A liver disorder in which the primary symptom is jaundice	h. quinquecuspid
______ 24.	Being 1/1000 of a volt	i. supratympanic
______ 25.	Situated above the tympanum	j. inframammary

You may now go on to Test 11.

SECTION 12

Miscellaneous Words and Medical Specialties

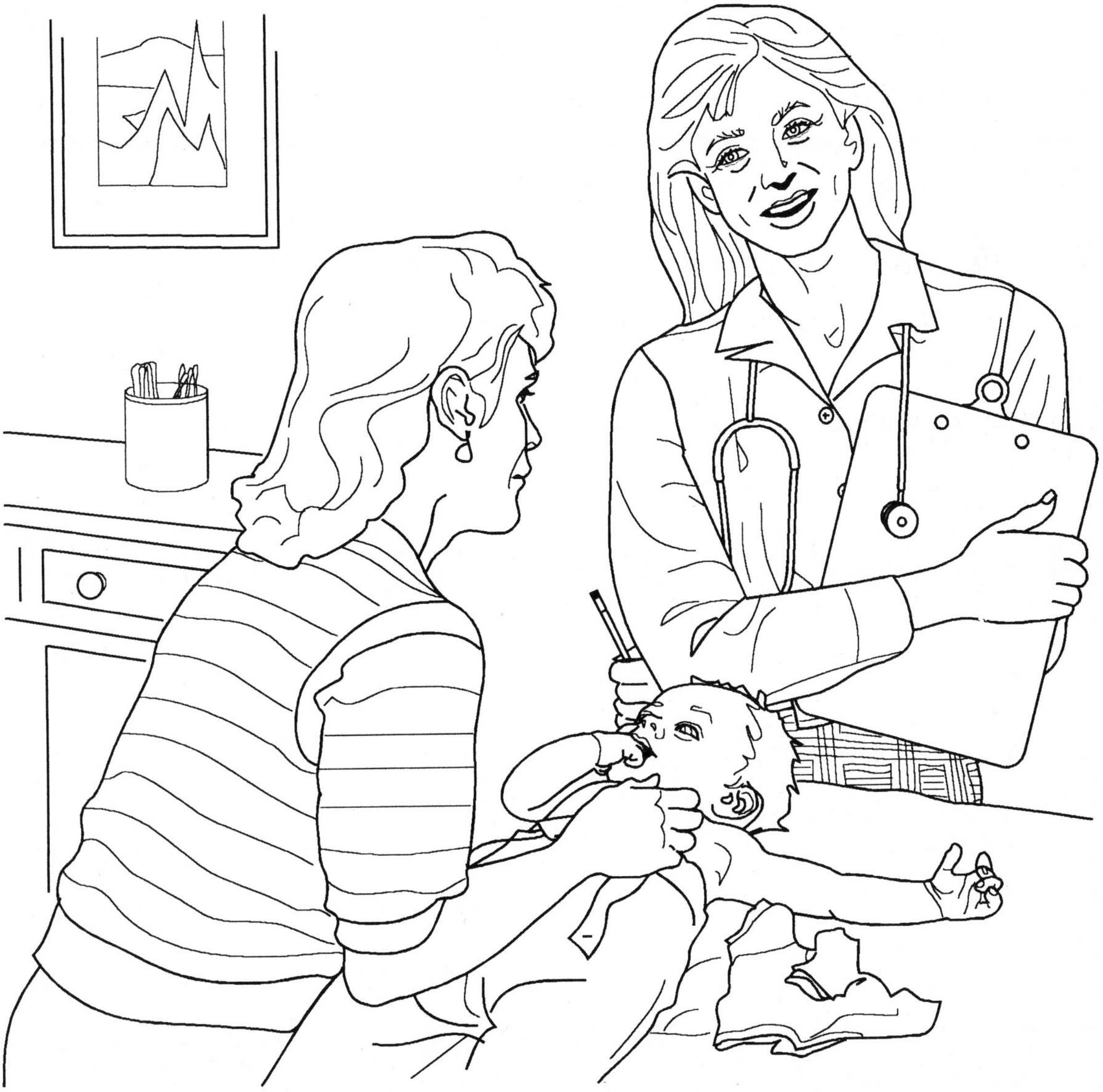

MISCELLANEOUS WORDS AND MEDICAL SPECIALTIES

Orientation

The following lessons make the student familiar with the medical specialties. Since any person working in the medical field will come into contact with these physicians on a daily basis, it is quite important that he or she recognize these specialties.

It is also important to realize the steps and time elements an individual spends to become a physician and specialist. The following is a brief chronological sequence of the steps it takes to become a medical specialist. First, a four year pre-med undergraduate program, followed by a four-year term in medical school. At this point, the individual serves a two to five year residency in the chosen specialty, i.e., internal medicine, radiology, etc.

After successful completion of a medical residency, some physicians undertake a postresidency fellowship in a subspecialty. The internist may choose cardiology or hematology-oncology among several sub-specialties. The general surgeon may elect a subspecialty of thoracic surgery or proctology.

A sound knowledge of these specialties and their function is essential to a person working in the medical field.

LESSON

56

Terminology Presentation

Miscellaneous Words

This lesson presents 18 miscellaneous words. Listen to the Lab Tape provided by your instructor, and you will hear the words presented in this lesson. Read the words as they are said, noticing spelling and pronunciation. The recording will tell you when the presentation for this lesson is completed and will give you any further instructions. Do not go on to the next recorded lesson until you have completed Lesson 56 and feel that you know the words and word parts that have been presented.

• • • ▶ *Start Audio*

WORD	WORD PART	DEFINITION	ANSWER
1. chyluria (ki-lu′re-ah)	chyl(i)- -uria	juice (digestive) urine	1. ________________
2. idiosyncrasy (id′e-o-sin′krah-se)	idi(o)- -syncrasy	self, one's own mixture, quality	2. ________________
3. pseudocyesis (soo′do-si-e′sis)	pseud(o)- -cyesis	false pregnancy	3. ________________
4. homogenesis (ho′mo-jen′e-sis)	hom(o)- -genesis	same producing	4. ________________
5. neoplasm (ne′o-plazm)	neo- -plasm	new formation	5. ________________
6. dyskinesia (dis′ki-ne′ze-ah)	dys- -kinesia	abnormal, painful movement	6. ________________
7. cryptorchidism (krip-tor′ki-dizm)	crypt(o)- orch(ido) -ism	hidden testes, testicle condition	7. ________________
8. pharmacologist (fahr′mah-kol′o-jist)	pharmac(o)- -logist	drug specialist	8. ________________
9. narcolepsy (nar′ko-lep′se)	narc(o)- -lepsy	numbness, sleep seizure	9. ________________
10. photoretinitis (fo′to-ret′i-ni′tis)	phot(o)- retin(o) -itis	light retina (of the eye) inflammation	10. ________________

11. rachiocentesis (ra′ke-o-sen-te′sis)	rachi(o)- -centesis	spine surgical puncture	**11.** ________
12. saprophyte (sap′ro-fit)	sapr(o)- -phyte	pus, decay plant, organism	**12.** ________
13. trachelodynia (tra′ke-lo-din′e-ah)	trachel(o)- -dynia	neck pain	**13.** ________
14. zoophobia (zo′o-fo′be-ah)	zo(o)- -phobia	animal fear	**14.** ________
15. crymodynia (kri′mo-din′e-ah)	crym(o)- -dynia	cold pain	**15.** ________
16. fasciotomy (fash′e-ot′o-me)	fasci(o)- -tomy	band incision, cutting into	**16.** ________
17. etiology (e′te-ol′o-je)	etio- -logy	cause study of, science of	**17.** ________
18. amblyopia (am′ble-o′pe-ah)	ambly- -opia	dull eye	**18.** ________

■ • • • *Stop Audio at Tone*

Study the 18 words and word parts for this lesson. Practice each word several times, checking your spelling and repeating the meaning to yourself. Listen to the recording and pronounce the words as many times as necessary. When you feel that you know the words and word parts well, you are ready to go on to the next step.

Use a sheet of paper to cover all columns except the Answer Column on the previous page. The words you have learned will be presented again on the recording. As each word is pronounced, write it in the space provided in the Answer Column.

• • • ▶ *Start Audio*

After stopping the tape player, check the words you have written against the words in the left-hand column. If any words are misspelled, practice writing them correctly. When you feel that you know and understand the words and word parts, go on to the Terminology Practice.

PRACTICE

____

____

____

____

Name ______________________ Date ______________ Errors ________

LESSON 56: TERMINOLOGY PRACTICE

Miscellaneous Words

Without looking at your previous work, write the word that is described by each definition.

DEFINITION	TERM
1. A congenital failure of the testes to descend into the scrotum	______________
2. Any new or abnormal growth	______________
3. Rheumatic pain coming on in cold or damp weather	______________
4. Lazy or dull eye	______________
5. Inflammation of the retina due to exposure to intense light	______________
6. Abnormal fear or dread of animals	______________
7. Spurious or false pregnancy	______________
8. Study of the cause of disease	______________
9. Reproduction by the same process each generation	______________
10. One who specializes in the study of the action of drugs	______________
11. Spinal (lumbar) puncture	______________
12. A habit or quality of body or mind peculiar to any individual	______________
13. Incision into fibrous tissue	______________
14. Presence of chyle in the urine	______________
15. Pain in the neck	______________
16. Difficult or painful movement	______________
17. An uncontrollable desire for sleep occurring at intervals	______________
18. An organism, such as bacteria, living upon decaying matter	______________

Check your answers against the word and definition lists on the first page of this lesson. If you have any errors, count them and write the number in the blank at the top of the page. Practice any missed or misspelled words in the space provided. Sign your work and give it to your instructor. You are now ready for the next lesson.

PRACTICE

LESSON

57

Terminology Presentation

Medical Specialties, Part 1

This lesson presents the names of 10 medical specialties and the corresponding specialists who work in these areas. As the names of the specialties are pronounced on the Lab Tape, read the list below, noticing the spelling and pronunciation of each. Practice the names and study the explanation of each specialty carefully. Repeat the recording as often as necessary.

• • • ▶ *Start Audio*

SPECIALTY	SPECIALIST

1. Anesthesiology (an′es-the′ze-ol′o-je) — Anesthesiologist (an′es-the′ze-ol′o-jist)

   Anesthesiology is the study and practice of administering anesthetic agents.

2. Dermatology (der′mah-tol′o-je) — Dermatologist (der′mah-tol′o-jist)

   Dermatology deals with the diagnosis and treatment of diseases of the skin.

3. Family Practice (Family Medicine) (fam′i-le prak′tis) — Family Practitioner (fam′i-le prak-tish′un-er)

   Family medicine concerns the diagnosis and treatment of disorders of all members of the family regardless of age or sex, on a continuing basis.

4. Obstetrics and Gynecology (ob-stet′riks) (gi′ne-kol′o-je) — Obstetrician and Gynecologist (ob′ste-trish′un) (gi′ne-kol′o-jist)

   Obstetrics deals with pregnancy, prenatal care, and childbirth and its aftermath; gynecology deals with disorders of women.

5. Ophthalmology (of′thal-mol′o-je) — Ophthalmologist (of′thal-mol′o-jist)

   This specialty deals with diseases of the eye. The ophthalmologist is a physician who deals with all areas involving the eye, as distinct from the optometrist who examines and tests eyes and treats visual defects with corrective lenses but is not a physician.

6. Physical Medicine and Rehabilitation (fiz′e-kal med′i-sin) — Physiatrist (fiz′e-at′rist)

   Physical medicine and rehabilitation deal with the diagnosis and treatment of diseases with the aid of physical agents such as heat, light, water, or mechanical apparatus. Exercise therapy and the use of braces are involved. The nonphysician in this area is known as a physical therapist.

7. Psychiatry and Neurology (si-ki'ah-tre) (nu-rol'o-je) — Psychiatrist and Neurologist (si-ki'ah-trist) (nu-rol'o-jist)

Psychiatry deals with functional disorders of the mind. Neurology deals with disorders of the nervous system caused by organic disease or injury.

8. Otolaryngology (o'to-lar'in-gol'o-je) — Otolaryngologist (o'to-lar'in-gol'o-jist)

This specialty involves the diagnosis and treatment of diseases of the ear, nose, and throat. Both surgical and nonsurgical techniques are employed.

9. Pathology (pah-thol'o-je) — Pathologist (pah-thol'o-jist)

The pathologist deals primarily with the diagnosis of disease. By studying the structural changes that have taken place, the pathologist can determine the cause of death.

10. Pediatrics (pe'de-at'riks) — Pediatrician (pe'de-ah'trish'un)

Pediatrics involves the diagnosis and treatment of diseases of children.

■ • • • *Stop Audio at Tone*

When you feel that you know the spelling, pronunciation, and meaning of each specialty and specialist thoroughly, go on to the Terminology Practice.

Name ________________________________ Date ____________________ Errors __________

LESSON 57: TERMINOLOGY PRACTICE

Medical Specialties, Part 1

Complete the sentences below with the names of the specialties and specialists.

1. ________________________ is the branch of medicine that treats disorders of the skin. The specialist is known as a(n) ________________________.

2. A division of medicine which studies and administers anesthetic agents is known as ________________________. The specialist is called a(n) ________________________.

3. A ________________________ deals with the diagnosis of diseases by studying structural changes in the body. This branch of medicine is called ________________________.

4. ________________________ is the branch of medicine treating disorders and diseases of children. The specialist is known as a(n) ________________________.

5. ________________________ and ________________________ are branches of medicine dealing with female disorders and pregnancy and childbirth. The specialists are known as ________________________ and ________________________.

6. The ________________________ is the specialist who treats disorders of the ear, nose, and throat. The specialty is called ________________________.

7. The ________________________ treats disorders of the eye. The specialty is known as ________________________.

8. The specialist using natural elements, such as heat and light, for treatment is known as a(n) ________________________. The branch of medicine is called ________________________.

9. The ______________________ and ______________________ deal with disorders of the nervous system and the mind. These branches of medicine are called ______________________ and ______________________.

10. The ______________ ______________ specializes in the diagnosis and treatment of all family members regardless of sex, on a continuing basis. The specialty is known as ______________ ______________.

Check your answers against the word and definition lists on the first page of this lesson. If you have any errors, count them and write the number in the blank at the top of the page. Practice any missed or misspelled words in the space provided. Sign your work and give it to your instructor. You are now ready for the next lesson.

PRACTICE

LESSON

58 Terminology Presentation

Medical Specialties, Part 2

This lesson presents the names of 10 medical specialties and the corresponding specialists who work in these areas. As the names of the specialties are pronounced on the Lab Tape, read the list below, noticing the spellings and pronunciation of each. Practice the names and study the explanation of each specialty carefully. Repeat the recording as often as necessary.

• • • ▸ *Start Audio*

SPECIALTY	SPECIALIST
1. Surgery (General Surgery) (sur′jer-e)	Surgeon (General Surgeon) (sur′jun)

Surgery is the branch of medicine which treats pathologic or traumatic conditions by operative procedures. The general surgeon operates for a variety of conditions, but some surgeons limit their work to just one.

2. Thoracic Surgery (tho-ras′ik)	Thoracic Surgeon (tho-ras′ik)

The thoracic surgeon deals with the diagnosis and treatment (mainly surgical) of disorders of the organs of the thoracic cavity, generally the heart and lungs.

3. Urology (u-rol′o-je)	Urologist (u-rol′o-jist)

Urology deals with the diagnosis and treatment of disorders and diseases of the urogenital system. Disorders of the urinary system of both men and women are treated by the urologist. Treatment of male genital disorders are common in this practice.

4. Proctology (Colon and Rectal Surgery) (prok-tol′o-je)	Proctologist (prok-tol′o-jist)

Diseases and disorders of the rectum and sigmoid colon are included under this heading. Treatment often involves surgery for such disorders as cancer, hemorrhoids, and anal fissures.

5. Plastic Surgery (plas′tik sur′jer-e)	Plastic Surgeon (plas′tik sur′jun)

Plastic surgery deals with the restoration or repair of defects of the human body. This repair often is accomplished by means of tissue grafting.

6. Orthopedic Surgery — Orthopedic Surgeon or Orthopedist
(or′tho-pe′dik) — (or′tho-pe′dist)

Orthopedic surgery is concerned with the treatment of musculoskeletal disorders. Surgery is often done to alleviate these conditions but nonsurgical techniques utilizing casts, braces, or strappings are sometimes used. Orthopedic is also spelled Orthopaedic, but the pronunciation remains the same.

7. Neurosurgery — Neurosurgeon
(nu′ro-sur′jer-e) — (nu′ro-sur′jun)

This branch of medicine deals with the diagnosis and mainly surgical treatment of diseases and disorders of the central nervous system (brain and spinal cord).

8. Radiology — Radiologist
(ra′de-ol′o-je) — (ra′de-ol′o-jist)

Radiology refers to the diagnostic and therapeutic use of radiant energy. Roentgen rays, commonly called x-rays, are a major tool in diagnosing disease. Cobalt and other types of energy are used in treating diseases such as cancer.

9. Nuclear Medicine
(nu′kle-ar)

This branch of medicine is concerned with the use of radionuclides in the diagnosis and treatment of disease.

10. Preventive Medicine
(pre-ven′tiv)

This branch of study and practice aims at the prevention of disease.

■ • • • *Stop Audio at Tone*

When you feel that you know the spelling, pronunciation, and meaning of each specialty and specialist thoroughly, go on to the Terminology Practice.

Name ______________________ Date ______________ Errors ________

LESSON 58: TERMINOLOGY PRACTICE

Medical Specialties, Part 2

Complete the sentences below with the names of the specialties and specialists.

1. ______________ ______________ is the branch of medicine dealing with the restoration or repair of injuries or defects of the human body. The specialist in this field is called a(n) ______________ ______________.

2. The ______________ is the specialist in using x-ray or roentgenography. This branch of medicine is called ______________.

3. ______________ deals with the diagnosis and treatment of disorders of the urinary tract. The specialist is called a(n) ______________.

4. A(n) ______________ treats, mainly with surgery, disorders of the central nervous system. This specialty is known as ______________ ______________.

5. A(n) ______________ ______________ diagnoses and surgically treats disorders of the organs of the thoracic cavity. The specialty is known as ______________ ______________.

6. ______________ is that branch of medicine dealing with disorders of the rectum and colon. The specialist is a(n) ______________.

7. The ______________ treats pathological conditions by operative procedures. This practice is known as ______________.

8. ______________ ______________ is the branch of medicine which aims at the prevention of disease.

9. The branch of medicine concerned with the use of radionuclides in the diagnosis and treatment of disease is known as ______________ ______________.

10. ____________________ ____________________ is the branch of medicine dealing with the treatment of bones, muscles, etc. The specialist is known as a(n) ____________________ ____________________ or a(n) ____________________.

Check your answers against the word and definition lists on the first page of this lesson. If you have any errors, count them and write the number in the blank at the top of the page. Practice any missed or misspelled words in the space provided. Sign your work and give it to your instructor. You are now ready for the next lesson.

PRACTICE

LESSON

59

Terminology Presentation

Medical Specialties, Part 3

This lesson presents the specialty of Internal Medicine and nine subspecialties and subspecialists. A physician may branch out from a Board Specialty and become what is known as a subspecialist.

• • • ▶ *Start Audio*

SPECIALTY	SPECIALIST
1. Internal Medicine (in-ter′nal med′i-sin)	Internist (in-ter′nist)

The internist diagnoses and treats disorders and diseases of the internal structures of the body.

2. Allergy and Immunology (al′er-je) (im′u-nol′o-je)	Allergist and Immunologist (al′er-jist) (im′u-nol′o-jist)

These specialties are concerned with the diagnosis and treatment of allergies and the body's resistance to disease.

3. Cardiology (kar-de-ol′o-je)	Cardiologist (kar-de-ol′o-jist)

The diagnosis and treatment of heart disorders is the Cardiologist's area of specialization.

4. Gastroenterology (gas′tro-en′ter-ol′o-je)	Gastroenterologist (gas′tro-en′ter-ol′o-jist)

The gastroenterologist deals with the diagnosis and treatment of diseases of the stomach and intestines.

5. Pulmonary Disease (pul′mo-ner′e)	Chest Specialist

The diagnosis and treatment of diseases of the chest or thorax is the concern of this specialist.

6. Endocrinology and Metabolism (en′do-kri-nol′o-je) (me-tab′o-lizm)	Endocrinologist (en′do-kri-nol′o-jist)

The endocrinologist studies the internally secreting glands and their effect on the body and its metabolism.

7. Hematology-Oncology (hem′ah-tol′o-je) (ong-kol′o-je)	Hematologist-Oncologist (hem′ah-tol′o-jist) (ong-kol′o-jist)

Hematology is the branch of medicine that treats the blood and blood-forming elements and oncology deals with tumors, primarily cancer.

8. Infectious Disease (Epidemiology) — Epidemiologist
(in-fek'shus) — (ep'i-de'me-ol'o-jist)

Epidemiology is the diagnosis and treatment of diseases capable of being communicated from one host to another.

9. Nephrology — Nephrologist
(ne-frol'o-je) — (ne-frol'o-jist)

The nephrologist diagnoses and treats diseases and disorders that involve the kidneys.

10. Rheumatology — Rheumatologist
(roo'mah-tol'o-je) — (roo'mah-tol'o-jist)

The science of rheumatism, a variety of disorders involving connective tissues (joints and related structures), is the area of this specialist.

■ • • • *Stop Audio at Tone*

When you feel that you know the spelling, pronunciation, and meaning of each specialty and specialist thoroughly, go on to the Terminology Practice.

Name ______________________ Date ______________ Errors ________

LESSON 59: TERMINOLOGY PRACTICE

Medical Specialties, Part 3

Complete the sentences below with the names of the specialties and specialists.

1. The ______________ and ______________ deal with the diagnosis and treatment of allergies and the body's resistance to disease. The specialties are known as ______________ and ______________.

2. A(n) ______________ deals with the diagnosis and treatment of diseases capable of being communicated from one host to another.

3. ______________ ______________ is the branch of medicine which deals with the diagnosis and treatment of the internal structures of the body. This specialist is known as a(n) ______________.

4. The ______________ specializes in the diagnosis and treatment of kidney disorders. The specialty is known as ______________.

5. ______________ and ______________ is the branch of medicine dealing with blood and blood-forming elements and cancer. The specialists in these areas are ______________ and ______________.

6. A(n) ______________ treats heart disorders. His or her specialty is known as ______________.

7. A(n) ______________ treats a variety of disorders of connective tissue (rheumatism). The specialty is ______________.

8. ______________ is the science of the diagnosis and treatment of diseases of the stomach and intestines. This specialist is known as a(n) ______________.

9. The specialty involved with the study of internally secreting glands is known as __________________________ and __________________________. The specialist is called a(n) __________________________.

10. __________________________ __________________________ is the branch of medicine that deals with the diagnosis and treatment of diseases of the chest or thorax. The specialist is called a(n) __________________________ __________________________.

Check your answers against the word and definition lists on the first page of this lesson. If you have any errors, count them and write the number in the blank at the top of the page. Practice any missed or misspelled words in the space provided. Sign your work and give it to your instructor. You are now ready for the next lesson.

PRACTICE

Name ________________ Date ________________ Errors ________

LESSON 60 — TERMINOLOGY REVIEW FOR TEST 12

This is a review of the words you have learned in the preceding four lessons.

Unlike the review for Test 11, the words are not written out for you. As each word is pronounced on the Lab Tape, write it in the appropriate numbered blank on the left, then write the appropriate definition in the space to the right.

• • • ▶ *Start Audio*

WORD	MEANING OR DEFINITION
1. ________________	________________
2. ________________	________________
3. ________________	________________
4. ________________	________________
5. ________________	________________
6. ________________	________________
7. ________________	________________

8. ______________________ ______________________________

____

____

9. ______________________ ______________________________

____

____

10. ______________________ ______________________________

____

____

11. ______________________ ______________________________

____

____

12. ______________________ ______________________________

____

____

13. ______________________ ______________________________

____

____

14. ______________________ ______________________________

____

____

15. ______________________ ______________________________

____

____

■ • • • *Stop Audio at Tone*

After all 15 words have been written, write the definition of each one. Use the Glossary or a dictionary to check your spellings and definitions. Practice the words on a separate sheet of paper, paying particular attention to any you missed or misspelled.

When you feel you know the words and definitions well, sign your work, indicate the number of errors, and turn your work in to your instructor. You are now ready for the Extra Credit Review (if your instructor assigns it) or Test 12.

Name ____________________ Date ____________ Errors ________

LESSON 60 EXTRA CREDIT REVIEW

This Extra Credit Review should be done at the discretion of your instructor. If you are instructed to complete this portion of the Review, turn it in to your instructor when you are finished.

PART A

Write the definition for the following 20 terms to the right of the given term.

TERM	DEFINITION
1. Dermatology	____________________
2. saprophyte	____________________
3. Ophthalmologist	____________________
4. Urology	____________________
5. Plastic Surgeon	____________________
6. idiosyncrasy	____________________
7. Otolaryngologist	____________________
8. Pathology	____________________
9. cryptorchidism	____________________
10. Rheumatology	____________________
11. neoplasm	____________________
12. Neurosurgeon	____________________
13. Internal Medicine	____________________
14. Pediatrician	____________________
15. Orthopedic Surgery	____________________
16. Anesthesiologist	____________________
17. chyluria	____________________
18. Obstetrician	____________________

19. Thoracic Surgeon ____________________

20. Psychiatry ____________________

PART B

Match the following definitions with the terms given. Place the correct letter of the definition to the left of the term.

TERM	DEFINITION
______ 21. pseudocyesis	a. diagnosis and treatment of diseases and disorders of the rectum and sigmoid colon
______ 22. Epidemiology	b. diagnosis and treatment of diseases and disorders of the urogenital system
______ 23. dyskinesis	c. diagnosis and treatment of diseases of the stomach and intestines
______ 24. Proctology	d. study of the causes of disease
______ 25. Nephrology	e. spurious or false pregnancy
______ 26. rachiocentesis	f. diagnosis and treatment of diseases and disorders of the kidneys
______ 27. Urology	g. diagnosis and treatment of diseases capable of being communicated from one host to another
______ 28. trachelodynia	h. spinal puncture
______ 29. Gastroenterology	i. pain in the neck
______ 30. etiology	j. difficult or painful movement

You may now go on to Test 12.

SECTION 13

Dental Terminology

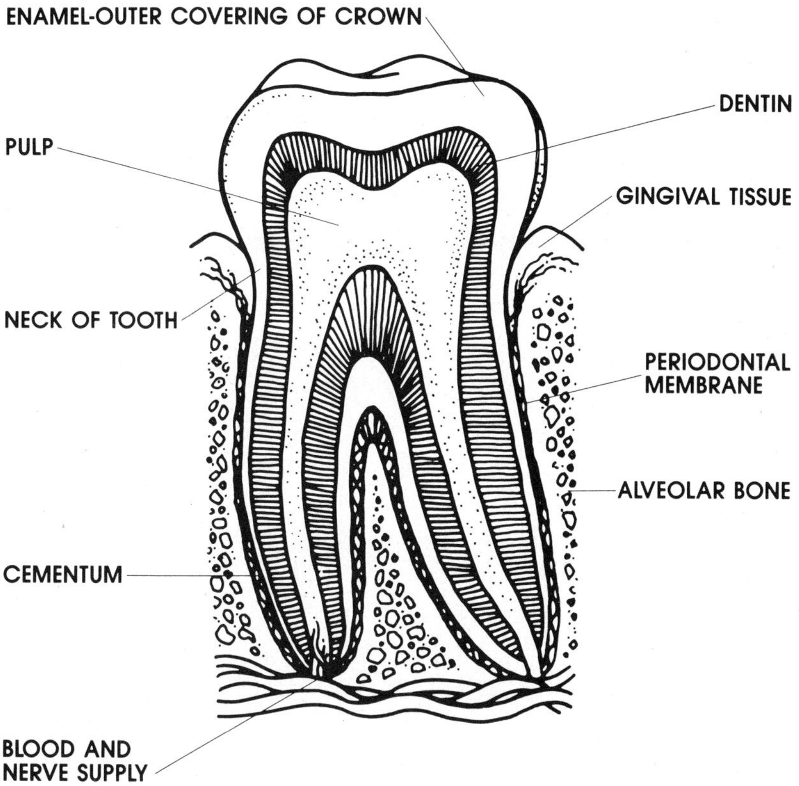
ENAMEL-OUTER COVERING OF CROWN
DENTIN
PULP
GINGIVAL TISSUE
NECK OF TOOTH
PERIODONTAL MEMBRANE
ALVEOLAR BONE
CEMENTUM
BLOOD AND NERVE SUPPLY

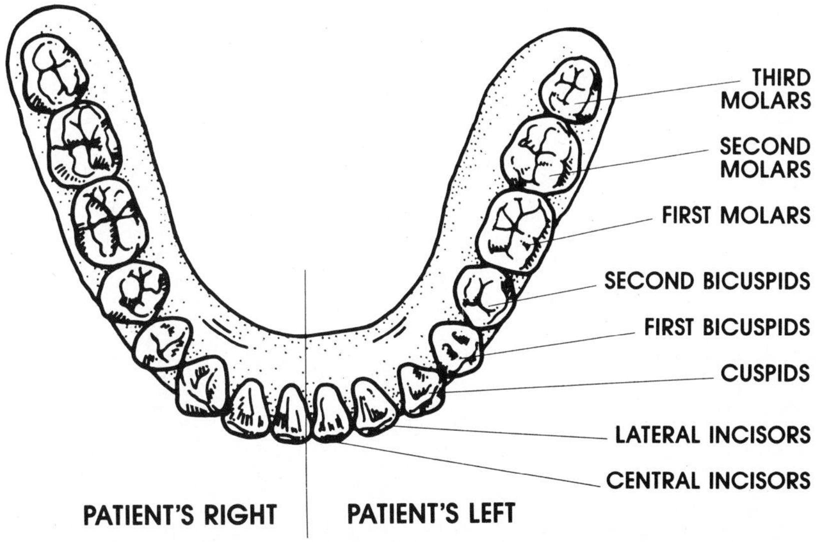
THIRD MOLARS
SECOND MOLARS
FIRST MOLARS
SECOND BICUSPIDS
FIRST BICUSPIDS
CUSPIDS
LATERAL INCISORS
CENTRAL INCISORS
PATIENT'S RIGHT
PATIENT'S LEFT

DENTAL TERMINOLOGY

Orientation

The mouth, which was also discussed in the digestive system, is the realm of the dental professional. Dental practitioners include dentists, dental assistants, dental hygienists, and dental technicians.

Each person has two sets of teeth, primary and secondary. There are 20 primary or "baby" teeth, ten upper and ten lower. These primary teeth are usually lost between six and twelve years of age. They are then replaced by the secondary or adult teeth of which there are 32 in most people. These are also known as permanent teeth. Third molars or "wisdom" teeth arrive somewhat later, usually by the age of 18.

A tooth is composed of the minerals calcium and phosphorus. The part of a tooth visible in the mouth is known as the crown. The gingival tissue (gums) surround the teeth. The surface of the crown is enamel. Inside the hard enamel shell of a tooth is the dentin. The central portion of a tooth is the pulp chamber, rich with passageways for vessels and nerves. At the base of the dentin is the root of the tooth which is covered by a thin material called cementum.

Teeth are named by their location in the jaw and by their function, for example, upper central incisor. An incisor is a cutting tooth, whereas a molar is a grinding tooth.

LESSON

61

Terminology Presentation

Dental Terminology, Part 1

Listen to the Lab Tape provided by your instructor, and you will hear the words presented in this lesson. Read the words as they are said, noticing spelling and pronunciation. The recording will tell you when the presentation for this lesson is completed and will give you any further instructions. Do not go on to the next recorded lesson until you have completed Lesson 61 and feel that you know the words and definitions that have been presented.

• • • ▶ *Start Audio*

	WORD	DEFINITION	ANSWER
1.	abrasion (ah-bra′zhun)	The wearing away or wearing down of teeth	1. ______________
2.	abutment (ah-but′ment)	Tooth that provides the point of anchorage for a bridge	2. ______________
3.	acrylic resins (ah-kril′ik rez′ins)	Plastic materials used in the fabrication of dentures and crowns	3. ______________
4.	alloy (al′loi)	The product formed as a result of combining two or more metals	4. ______________
5.	amalgam (ah-mal′gam)	An alloy used to fill teeth containing mercury, silver, and tin	5. ______________
6.	appliance (ah-pli′ans)	A device worn by a dental patient during the course of treatment	6. ______________
7.	articulate (ar-tik′u-lat)	To unite the teeth of one arch in the proper position with the teeth of the opposing arch	7. ______________
8.	articulator (ar-tik′u-la′tor)	An instrument for holding the casts of jaws or teeth in the proper relationship to one another	8. ______________
9.	attrition (ah-trish′un)	Wearing down the surfaces of teeth by chewing	9. ______________
10.	bacterial plaque (bak-te′re-al plak)	A film-like covering on the teeth.	10. ______________

11. baseplate (bas′plat)	A sheet of wax or metal that is used for trial denture setups	**11.** ______	
12. bicuspids (bi-cus′pids)	Teeth with two cusps, situated between cuspids and molars	**12.** ______	
13. bruxism (bruk′sizm)	The clenching or grinding of the teeth	**13.** ______	
14. burnishing (ber′nish-ing)	Polishing by friction	**14.** ______	
15. caries (kar′ez)	Decay of tooth structure	**15.** ______	

■ • • • *Stop Audio at Tone*

Study the 15 words for this lesson. Practice each word several times, checking your spelling and repeating the meaning to yourself. Listen to the recording and pronounce the words as many times as necessary. When you feel that you know the words well, you are ready to go on to the next step.

Use a sheet of paper to cover all columns except the Answer Column on the previous page. The words you have learned will be presented again on the recording. As each word is pronounced, write it in the space provided in the Answer Column.

• • • ▶ *Start Audio*

After stopping the tape player, check the words you have written against the words in the left-hand column. If any words are misspelled, practice writing them correctly. When you feel that you know and understand the words and definitions, go on to the Terminology Practice.

PRACTICE

Name ______________________ Date ______________ Errors ________

LESSON 61: TERMINOLOGY PRACTICE

Dental Terminology, Part 1

Without looking at your previous work, write the word that is described by each definition.

DEFINITION	TERM
1. An alloy used to fill teeth containing mercury, silver, and tin	________________
2. An instrument for holding the casts of jaws or teeth in the proper relationship to one another	________________
3. Decay of tooth structure	________________
4. The wearing away or wearing down of teeth	________________
5. Teeth with two cusps, situated between cuspids and molars	________________
6. The product formed as a result of combining two or more metals	________________
7. A film-like covering on the teeth	________________
8. Tooth that provides the point of anchorage for a bridge	________________
9. A device worn by a dental patient during the course of treatment	________________
10. The clenching or grinding of teeth	________________
11. Plastic material used in the fabrication of dentures and crowns	________________
12. Polishing by friction	________________
13. Wearing down of the surfaces of teeth by chewing	________________
14. A sheet of wax or metal that is used for trial dental setups	________________
15. To unite the teeth of one arch in the proper position with the teeth of the opposing arch	________________

Check your answers against the word and definition lists on the first page of this lesson. If you have any errors, count them and write the number in the blank at the top of the page. Practice any missed or misspelled words in the space provided. Sign your work and give it to your instructor. You are now ready for the next lesson.

PRACTICE

LESSON 62

Terminology Presentation

Dental Terminology, Part 2

Listen to the Lab Tape provided by your instructor, and you will hear the words presented in this lesson. Read the words as they are said, noticing spelling and pronunciation. The recording will tell you when the presentation for this lesson is completed and will give you any further instructions. Do not go on to the next recorded lesson until you have completed Lesson 62 and feel that you know the words and definitions that have been presented.

• • • ▸ *Start Audio*

WORD	DEFINITION	ANSWER
1. contact point (kon′takt point)	The area of a tooth's surface that touches a neighboring tooth	1. ______________
2. crown (krown)	The portion of a tooth that is covered by enamel and projects from the gum	2. ______________
3. crown and bridge (krown brij)	The branch of dentistry concerned with the replacement of natural tooth structures with dental prostheses	3. ______________
4. cuspid (kus′pid)	A tooth with one point or cusp	4. ______________
5. dental arch (den′tal arch)	The curved structure of natural dentition	5. ______________
6. dental hygienist (den′tal hi-je′nist)	A person trained in the art of dental prophylaxis	6. ______________
7. dental technician (den′tal tek-nish′an)	A person trained in the fabrication of dental appliances or devices (dentures, etc.)	7. ______________
8. dentin (den′tin)	The tissue that constitutes the chief substance of a tooth	8. ______________
9. denture (den′chur)	An artificial substitute for missing natural teeth	9. ______________
10. edentulous (e-den′tu-lus)	Having no teeth	10. ______________

11. enamel (en-am'el)	The hard tissue that covers the dentin of the crown portion of a tooth	**11.** ______________
12. endodontics (en'do-don'tiks)	The branch of dentistry concerned with cause, prevention, diagnosis, and treatment of injuries or diseases of the teeth	**12.** ______________
13. exodontics (ek'so-don'tiks)	The branch of dentistry concerned with the extraction or removal of teeth	**13.** ______________
14. extraction (eks-trak'shun)	The surgical removal of a tooth	**14.** ______________
15. fluoridation (floo'or-i-da'shun)	The addition of fluoride to a community water supply to control dental caries	**15.** ______________

■ • • • *Stop Audio at Tone*

Study the 15 words for this lesson. Practice each word several times, checking your spelling and repeating the meaning to yourself. Listen to the recording and pronounce the words as many times as necessary. When you feel that you know the words well, you are ready to go on to the next step.

Use a sheet of paper to cover all columns except the Answer Column on the previous page. The words you have learned will be presented again on the recording. As each word is pronounced, write it in the space provided in the Answer Column.

• • • ▸ *Start Audio*

After stopping the tape player, check the words you have written against the words in the left-hand column. If any words are misspelled, practice writing them correctly. When you feel that you know and understand the words and definitions, go on to the Terminology Practice.

PRACTICE

____

____

____

____

____

____

____

Name ______________________ Date ______________ Errors ________

LESSON 62: TERMINOLOGY PRACTICE

Dental Terminology, Part 2

Without looking at your previous work, write the word that is described by each definition.

DEFINITION	TERM
1. The curved structure of natural dentition	________
2. The surgical removal of a tooth	________
3. The area of a tooth's surface that touches a neighboring tooth	________
4. The addition of fluoride to a community water supply to control dental caries	________
5. The portion of a tooth that is covered by enamel and projects from the gum	________
6. A person trained in the fabrication of dental appliances or devices (dentures, etc.)	________
7. A tooth with one point or cusp	________
8. The branch of dentistry concerned with cause, prevention, diagnosis, and treatment of injuries or diseases of the teeth	________
9. Having no teeth	________
10. The hard tissue that covers the dentin of the crown portion of a tooth	________
11. The branch of dentistry concerned with the extraction or removal of teeth	________
12. A person trained in the art of dental prophylaxis	________
13. The branch of dentistry concerned with the replacement of natural tooth structures with dental prostheses	________
14. The tissue that constitutes the chief substance of a tooth	________
15. An artificial substitute for missing natural teeth	________

Check your answers against the word and definition lists on the first page of this lesson. If you have any errors, count them and write the number in the blank at the top of the page. Practice any missed or misspelled words in the space provided. Sign your work and give it to your instructor. You are now ready for the next lesson.

PRACTICE

LESSON
63

Terminology Presentation

Dental Terminology, Part 3

Listen to the Lab Tape provided by your instructor, and you will hear the words presented in this lesson. Read the words as they are said, noticing spelling and pronunciation. The recording will tell you when the presentation for this lesson is completed and will give you any further instructions. Do not go on to the next recorded lesson until you have completed Lesson 63 and feel that you know the words and definitions that have been presented.

• • • ▶ *Start Audio*

WORD	DEFINITION	ANSWER
1. fluoride, topical (floo′o-rid top′e-kal)	The direct application of fluoride to the teeth	1. ________
2. frenum, labial (fre′num la′be-al) frenum, lingual (ling′gwal)	The band of tissue inside the lip The band of tissue under the tongue	2. ________
3. gingiva (jin′ji-vah)	The tissue enveloping the tooth sockets (the gums)	3. ________
4. impacted tooth (im-pakt′ed)	A tooth embedded in the soft or bony tissues of the jaw that has not totally or partially come through	4. ________
5. incisor (in-si′zer)	A tooth with a cutting edge	5. ________
6. inlay, dental (in′la den′tal)	A cast restoration carved to replace the missing part of a tooth	6. ________
7. jacket (jak′et)	A crown fabricated of porcelain or metal; often called a “cap”	7. ________
8. malar (ma′lar)	Referring to the cheek or cheekbone	8. ________
9. malocclusion (mal′o-kloo′zhun)	A deviation of normal contact of the upper and lower jaw	9. ________
10. mandible (man′di-bl)	The lower jawbone	10. ________

11. mastication (mas′ti-ka′shun)	The act or process of chewing	**11.** ______________
12. maxilla (mak-sil′ah)	The upper jawbone	**12.** ______________
13. molar (mo′lar)	A grinding tooth	**13.** ______________
14. occlusal surface (o-kloo′zal)	The chewing or grinding surface of a tooth	**14.** ______________
15. occlusion (o-kloo′zhun)	The natural closure and fitting together of the upper and lower teeth	**15.** ______________

■ • • • *Stop Audio at Tone*

Study the 15 words for this lesson. Practice each word several times, checking your spelling and repeating the meaning to yourself. Listen to the recording and pronounce the words as many times as necessary. When you feel that you know the words well, you are ready to go on to the next step.

Use a sheet of paper to cover all columns except the Answer Column on the previous page. The words you have learned will be presented again on the recording. As each word is pronounced, write it in the space provided in the Answer Column.

• • • ▸ *Start Audio*

After stopping the tape player, check the words you have written against the words in the left-hand column. If any words are misspelled, practice writing them correctly. When you feel that you know and understand the words and definitions, go on to the Terminology Practice.

PRACTICE

Name ______________________ Date ______________ Errors ________

LESSON 63: TERMINOLOGY PRACTICE
Dental Terminology, Part 3

Without looking at your previous work, write the word that is described by each definition.

DEFINITION	TERM
1. The tissue enveloping the tooth sockets (the gums)	______________
2. A cast restoration carved to replace the missing part of a tooth	______________
3. Referring to the cheek or cheekbone	______________
4. The direct application of fluoride to the teeth	______________
5. The lower jawbone	______________
6. The natural closure and fitting together of the upper and lower teeth	______________
7. A deviation of normal contact of the upper and lower teeth	______________
8. The band of tissue inside the lip	______________
9. A tooth embedded in the soft or bony tissue of the jaw that has not totally or partially come through	______________
10. The chewing or grinding surface of a tooth	______________
11. A grinding tooth	______________
12. The act or process of chewing	______________
13. A crown fabricated of porcelain or metal; often called a "cap"	______________
14. A tooth with a cutting edge	______________
15. The upper jawbone	______________

Check your answers against the word and definition lists on the first page of this lesson. If you have any errors, count them and write the number in the blank at the top of the page. Practice any missed or misspelled words on the next page. Sign your work and give it to your instructor. You are now ready for the next lesson.

PRACTICE

LESSON

64

Terminology Presentation

Dental Terminology, Part 4

Listen to the Lab Tape provided by your instructor, and you will hear the words presented in this lesson. Read the words as they are said, noticing spelling and pronunciation. The recording will tell you when the presentation for this lesson is completed and will give you any further instructions. Do not go on to the next recorded lesson until you have completed Lesson 64 and feel that you know the words and definitions that have been presented.

• • • ▸ *Start Audio*

WORD	DEFINITION	ANSWER
1. oral pathology (o′ral pah-thol′o-je)	The branch of dentistry concerned with diseases of the teeth and mouth	1. ______
2. oral surgery (o′ral sur′jer-e)	The branch of dentistry involving operative procedures of the teeth and mouth	2. ______
3. orthodontics (or′tho-don′tiks)	The branch of dentistry that deals with the prevention and correction of irregularities of the teeth and malocclusion	3. ______
4. palate (pal′at)	The roof of the mouth	4. ______
5. pedodontics (pe-do-don′tiks)	The branch of dentistry that treats dental conditions in children	5. ______
6. permanent teeth (per′mah-nent teeth)	The teeth of adults	6. ______
7. pontic (pon′tik)	The portion of a dental bridge that replaces a missing tooth	7. ______
8. prosthesis (pros-the′sis)	The replacement of part of the body by an artificial part such as a denture	8. ______
9. prosthodontics (pros′tho-don′tiks)	Dentistry that deals with the replacement of natural teeth with prosthetics	9. ______

10.	pulp (pulp)	The soft tissue that fills the inside of teeth	10. ______________
11.	root (root)	The portion of a tooth that is in its socket	11. ______________
12.	root canal (root kah-nal′)	The space within the root of a tooth containing the pulp	12. ______________
13.	supernumerary tooth (soo′per-nu′mer-ar′e)	A tooth in excess of the regular number	13. ______________
14.	temporomandibular joint (tem′po-ro-man-dib′u-lar)	The joint, just ahead of the ear, which swings the lower jaw open	14. ______________
15.	zygomatic arch (zi′go-mat′ik)	The "cheekbone"	15. ______________

■ • • • *Stop Audio at Tone*

Study the 15 words for this lesson. Practice each word several times, checking your spelling and repeating the meaning to yourself. Listen to the recording and pronounce the words as many times as necessary. When you feel that you know the words well, you are ready to go on to the next step.

Use a sheet of paper to cover all columns except the Answer Column on the previous page. The words you have learned will be presented again on the recording. As each word is pronounced, write it in the space provided in the Answer Column.

• • • ▶ *Start Audio*

After stopping the tape player, check the words you have written against the words in the left-hand column. If any words are misspelled, practice writing them correctly. When you feel that you know and understand the words and definitions, go on to the Terminology Practice.

PRACTICE

____

____

____

____

____

____

____

____

Name ______________________ Date ______________ Errors ________

LESSON 64: TERMINOLOGY PRACTICE

Dental Terminology, Part 4

Without looking at your previous work, write the word that is described by each definition.

DEFINITION	TERM
1. The portion of a dental bridge that replaces a missing tooth	______________
2. Dentistry that deals with the replacement of natural teeth with prosthetics	______________
3. The soft tissue that fills the inside of teeth	______________
4. The roof of the mouth	______________
5. The branch of dentistry concerned with diseases of the teeth and mouth	______________
6. The portion of a tooth that is fixed in its socket	______________
7. The space within the root of a tooth containing the pulp	______________
8. The branch of dentistry concerned with operative procedures of the teeth and mouth	______________
9. The branch of dentistry that deals with dental conditions in children	______________
10. The joint, just ahead of the ear, which swings the lower jaw open	______________
11. The "cheekbone"	______________
12. The teeth of adults	______________
13. A tooth in excess of the regular number	______________
14. The replacement of part of the body by an artificial part such as a denture	______________
15. The branch of dentistry that deals with the prenvention and correction of irregularities of teeth and malocclusion	______________

Check your answers against the word and definition lists on the first page of this lesson. If you have any errors, count them and write the number in the blank at the top of the page. Practice any missed or misspelled words in the space provided. Sign your work and give it to your instructor. You are now ready for the next lesson.

PRACTICE

Name ______________________ Date ______________ Errors ________

LESSON 65 | TERMINOLOGY REVIEW FOR TEST 13

This is a review of the word parts you have learned in the preceding four lessons. As each word is pronounced on the Lab Tape, write the appropriate definition in the space to the right.

• • • ▸ *Start Audio*

WORD	DEFINITION
1. **articulate** (ar-tik′u-lat)	
2. edentulous (e-den′tu-lus)	
3. frenum, lingual (fre′num ling′gwal)	
4. incisor (in-si′zer)	
5. temporomandibular joint (tem′po-ro-man-dib′u-lar)	
6. pedodontics (pe-do-don′tiks)	
7. bruxism (bruk′sizm)	
8. gingiva (jin′ji-vah)	
9. molar (mo′lar)	
10. orthodontics (or′tho-don′tiks)	
11. prosthesis (pros-the′sis)	
12. malar (ma′lar)	
13. exodontics (ek′so-don′tiks)	

14. cuspid
(kus'pid) ____
____

15. amalgam
(ah-mal'gam) ____
____

■ • • • *Stop Audio at Tone*

After all 15 definitions have been written, use your book or a dictionary to check your spellings and definitions. Practice the words on a separate sheet of paper, paying particular attention to any you missed or misspelled.

When you feel you know the words and definitions well, sign your work, indicate the number of errors, and turn your work in to your instructor. You are now ready for the Extra Credit Review (if your instructor assigns it) or Test 13.

Name ______________________ Date ______________ Errors ________

LESSON 65 — EXTRA CREDIT REVIEW

This Extra Credit Review should be done at the discretion of your instructor. If you are instructed to complete this portion of the Review, turn it in to your instructor when you are finished.

PART A

Match the following terms with the definitions given. Place the correct letter of the term to the left of the definition.

DEFINITION

______ 1. The clenching or grinding of the teeth

______ 2. A tooth with one point or cusp

______ 3. Referring to the cheekbone

______ 4. The tissue enveloping the tooth socket (the gums)

______ 5. The branch of dentistry concerned with the extraction of teeth

______ 6. To unite the teeth of one arch in the proper position with the teeth of the opposing arch

______ 7. An alloy used to fill teeth containing mercury, tin, and silver

______ 8. Without teeth

______ 9. The joint, just ahead of the ear, which swings the lower jaw open

______ 10. The branch of dentistry that treats dental conditions in children

______ 11. A grinding tooth

______ 12. The replacement of part of the body by an artificial part such as a denture

______ 13. A tooth with a cutting edge

______ 14. The band of tissue under the tongue

______ 15. The branch of dentistry that deals with the prevention of irregularities of teeth and malocclusion

TERM

a. temporomandibular joint
b. amalgam
c. prosthesis
d. pedodontics
e. bruxism
f. frenum, lingual
g. gingiva
h. cuspid
i. malar
j. incisor
k. orthodontics
l. articulate
m. exodontics
n. molar
o. edentulous

PART B

Match the following definitions with the terms given. Place the correct letter of the definition to the left of the term.

TERM

______ **16.** prosthodontics

______ **17.** zygomatic arch

______ **18.** dentin

______ **19.** abutment

______ **20.** supernumerary tooth

______ **21.** bacterial plaque

______ **22.** occlusal surface

______ **23.** pontic

______ **24.** mandible

______ **25.** maxilla

DEFINITION

a. the lower jawbone
b. a film-like covering of the teeth
c. dentistry that deals with the replacement of natural teeth with prosthetics
d. the upper jawbone
e. the "cheekbone"
f. the portion of a dental bridge that replaces a missing tooth
g. the tissue that constitutes the chief substance of a tooth
h. the tooth that provides that point of anchorage for a bridge
i. the chewing or grinding surface of a tooth
j. a tooth in excess of the regular number

You may now go on to Test 13.

SECTION

14 Common Drugs

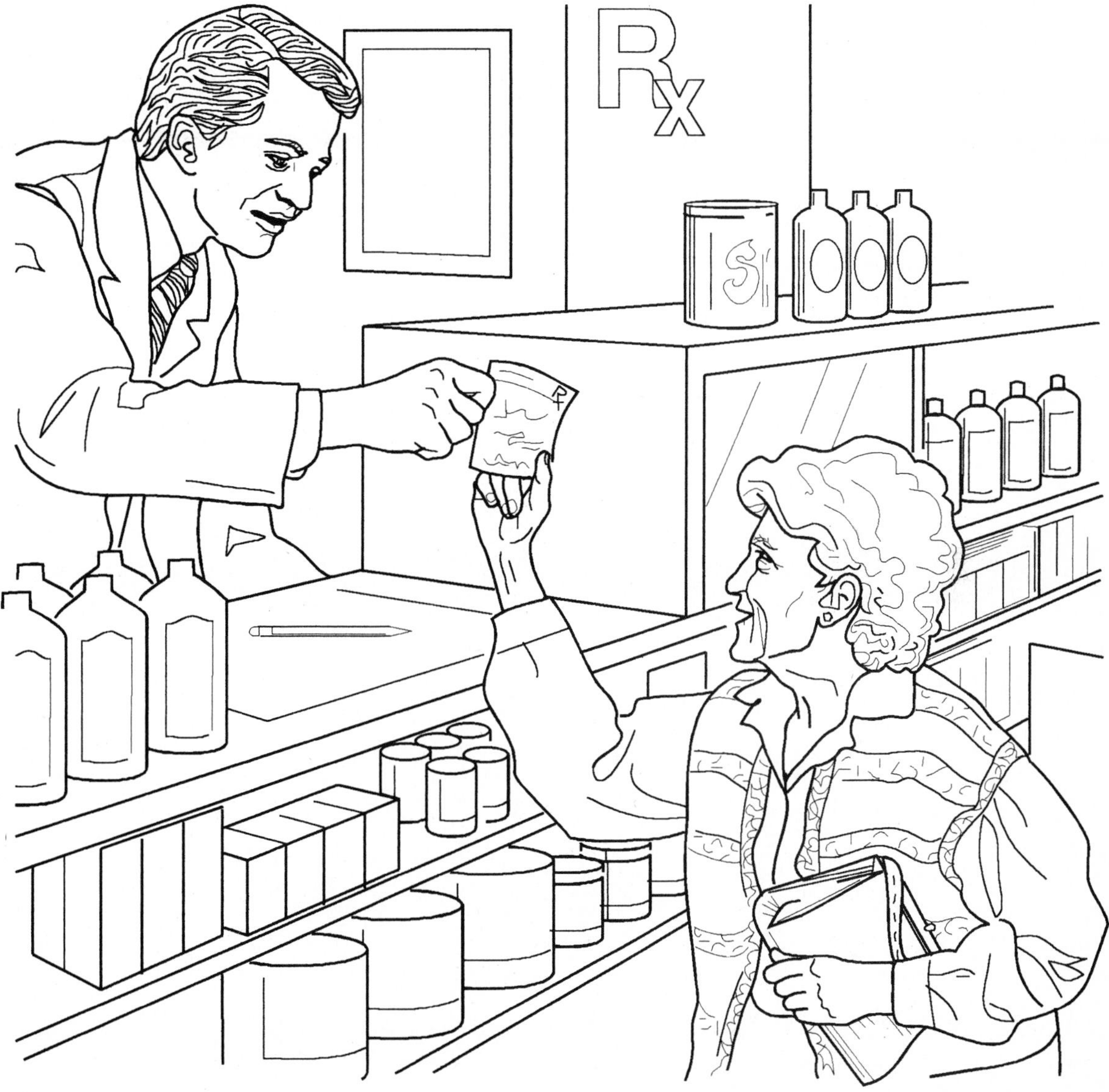

COMMON DRUGS

Orientation

This section follows the anatomic listing of systems of the body, i.e., cardiovascular, respiratory, etc., in presenting some common drugs prescribed for symptoms and disorders of the indicated system.

The intention of the author is to provide you with a brief definition of the drug, indicating the reason a given drug is prescribed. When possible, we have given either the generic or brand name of each drug.

If you wish more information about a given drug, it is suggested that you consult a current edition of the *Physicians' Desk Reference*, published by Medical Economics Company.

LESSON

66

Terminology Presentation

Drugs: Cardiovascular and Musculoskeletal Systems

Listen to the Lab Tape provided by your instructor, and you will hear the words presented in this lesson. Read the words as they are said, noticing spelling and pronunciation. The recording will tell you when the presentation for this lesson is completed and will give you any further instructions. Do not go on to the next recorded lesson until you have completed Lesson 66 and feel that you know the words that have been presented.

• • • ▶ ***Start Audio***

WORD	DEFINITION	ANSWER
1. digoxin (di-jok′sin)	The generic name of a drug which increases the contractions of the heart	1. ________
2. Mevacor (Mev-a-kor′)	Brand name for the generic drug lovastatin, used for lowering elevated serum cholesterol	2. ________
3. captopril (kap′to-pril)	Generic name for Capoten, a drug prescribed for high blood pressure in patients who have normal kidney function	3. ________
4. Vasotec (Vas′o-tek)	Brand name for the drug enalapril maleate, used in the treatment of high blood pressure	4. ________
5. propranolol (pro-pran′o-lol)	The generic name for Inderal, a potent drug which is prescribed for various heart conditions such as angina pectoris	5. ________
6. quinidine (kwin′i-din)	The generic name for Quinaglute, used to increase the contractability of the heart muscle. Also used to treat irregular rhythm of the heart	6. ________
7. Aldactazide (Al-dak′tah-zid)	Brand name for the generic drug spironolactone, used to treat high blood pressure and water accumulation in body tissue	7. ________
8. nitroglycerin (ni-tro-glis′er-in)	The generic name of a drug used to treat attacks of angina pectoris that are often present in various forms of heart disease. Brand names include Nitro-Dur II, Nitrobid and Nitrospan	8. ________

9.	ibuprofen (i-bu-pro'fen)	The generic name for Rufen or Motrin, prescribed as a pain reliever	9. ____________
10.	Flexeril (Flek'ser-il)	Brand name for the generic drug cyclobenzaprine, used for the relief of muscle spasms or stiffness	10. ____________
11.	prednisone (pred'ni-zon)	The generic name of a drug prescribed as an antiinflammatory agent	11. ____________
12.	Quinamm (Qwin'am)	Brand name for quinine sulfate, prescribed for nocturnal muscle cramps	12. ____________
13.	Plaquenil (Plak'kwin-il)	Brand name for the generic drug Hydroxychloroquine sulfate, prescribed for the treatment of acute or chronic rheumatoid arthritis and other disorders	13. ____________
14.	Voltaren (Vol'tah-ren)	Brand name for the generic drug diclofenac sodium, prescribed for the relief of acute and chronic symptoms of arthritis	14. ____________
15.	allopurinol (al-o-pu-ri-nol)	The generic name for Zyloprim, prescribed for the treatment of gout	15. ____________

■ • • • *Stop Audio at Tone*

Study the 15 words for this lesson. Practice each word several times, checking your spelling and repeating the meaning to yourself. Listen to the recording and pronounce the words as many times as necessary. When you feel that you know the words well, you are ready to go on to the next step.

Use a sheet of paper to cover all columns except the Answer Column on the previous page. The words you have learned will be presented again on the recording. As each word is pronounced, write it in the space provided in the Answer Column.

• • • ▶ *Start Audio*

After stopping the tape player, check the words you have written against the words in the left-hand column. If any words are misspelled, practice writing them correctly. When you feel that you know and understand the words, go on to the Terminology Practice.

PRACTICE

____

____

____

____

Name ______________________ Date ______________ Errors ________

LESSON 66: TERMINOLOGY PRACTICE

Drugs: Cardiovascular and Musculoskeletal Systems

Without looking at your previous work, write the word that is described by each definition. Since many of the drugs in this section have similar uses, the first letter of the drug matching the definition is given.

DEFINITION	TERM
1. Brand name for the drug enalapril maleate used in the treatment of high blood pressure	V __________
2. The generic name of a drug prescribed as an antiinflammatory agent	p __________
3. The generic name of a drug used to treat attacks of angina pectoris that are often present in various forms of heart disease. Brand names include Nitro-Dur II, Nitrospan and Nitro-bid	n __________
4. The generic name of a drug which increases the contractions of the heart	d __________
5. Brand name for the generic drug cyclobenzaprine, used for the relief of muscle spasms or stiffness	F __________
6. The generic name for Zyloprim, prescribed for the treatment of gout	a __________
7. The generic name for Quinaglute, used to increase the contractability of the heart muscle. Also used to treat irregular rhythm of the heart	q __________
8. Brand name for the generic drug diclofenac sodium, prescribed for the relief of acute and chronic symptoms of arthritis	V __________
9. Brand name for the generic drug lovastatin, used for lowering elevated serum cholesterol	M __________
10. Brand name for quinine sulfate, prescribed for nocturnal leg muscle cramps	Q __________
11. The generic name for Rufen or Motrin, prescribed as a pain reliever	i __________
12. The generic name for Inderal, a potent drug which is prescribed for various heart conditions such as angina pectoris	p __________
13. Brand name for the drug spironolactone, used to treat high blood pressure and water accumulation in body tissue	A __________

14. Generic name for Capoten, a drug prescribed for high blood pressure in patients who have normal kidney function — c ____________________

15. Brand name for the generic drug hydroxychloroquine sulfate, prescribed for the treatment of acute or chronic rheumatoid arthritis and other disorders — P ____________________

Check your answers against the word and definition lists on the first page of this lesson. If you have any errors, count them and write the number in the blank at the top of the page. Practice any missed or misspelled words in the space provided. Sign your work and give it to your instructor. You are now ready for the next lesson.

PRACTICE

LESSON

67

Terminology Presentation

Drugs: Integumentary and Genitourinary Systems

Listen to the Lab Tape provided by your instructor, and you will hear the words presented in this lesson. Read the words as they are said, noticing spelling and pronunciation. The recording will tell you when the presentation for this lesson is completed and will give you any further instructions. Do not go on to the next recorded lesson until you feel that you know the words that have been presented.

• • • ▸ *Start Audio*

WORD	DEFINITION	ANSWER
1. hydrocortisone (hi-dro-kor′ti-zon)	The generic name of a drug prescribed for several skin problems characterized by itching, swelling, redness, etc.	1. ________
2. Retin-A (Ret′in-a)	Brand name for the generic drug tretinoin, used in the treatment of some kinds of acne	2. ________
3. Accutane (Ak′u-tan)	Brand name for the generic drug isotretinoin, prescribed for patients with severe acne	3. ________
4. Mycolog (Mi′ko-log)	Brand name for the generic drug nystatin and neomycin sulfate, used for the control of dermatitis	4. ________
5. Lotrimin (Lot′ri-min)	Brand name for clotrimazole, prescribed as an antifungal agent in skin infections	5. ________
6. Zovirax (Zov′i-raks)	Brand name for the generic drug acyclovir, used in the treatment of genital herpes	6. ________
7. Diprolene (Di-pro′len)	Brand name for the generic drug betamethasone dipropionate, prescribed to relieve inflammation, itching and swelling of the skin	7. ________
8. Pyridium (Pi-rid′e-um)	Brand name for the generic drug phenozapyridine hydrochloride, prescribed for the relief of urinary pain, urgency, frequency, etc.	8. ________
9. Septra (Sep′trah)	Brand name of the generic drug trimethoprim sulfamethoxazole, used in the treatment of types of urinary infection	9. ________

10. Macrodantin (Mak′ro-dan-tin)	Brand name for the generic drug nitrofurantoin macrocrystals, prescribed as an antibacterial agent in urinary tract infections	10. ________
11. Urecholine (U′rek-o-len)	Brand name for bethanechol chloride, used for the treatment of postoperative and postpartum nonobstructive urinary retention	11. ________
12. Cipro (Sip′ro)	The brand name of the generic drug ciprofloxacin, an antibacterial agent used to treat a variety of infections	12. ________
13. Ditropan (Di′tro-pan)	Brand name for oxybutynin chloride, which is prescribed for the relief of symptoms of urinary instability	13. ________
14. Kwell (Kwel)	Brand name for the generic drug lindane, used for the treatment of scabies	14. ________
15. Azo Gantrisin (Azo-gant′ri-sin)	Brand name for the generic drug sulfisoxazole, which is prescribed for the treatment of infections of the urinary tract	15. ________

■ • • • *Stop Audio at Tone*

Study the 15 words for this lesson. Practice each word several times, checking your spelling and repeating the meaning to yourself. Listen to the recording and pronounce the words as many times as necessary. When you feel that you know the words well, you are ready to go on to the next step.

Use a sheet of paper to cover all columns except the Answer Column on the previous page. The words you have learned will be presented again on the recording. As each word is pronounced, write it in the space provided in the Answer Column.

• • • ▶ *Start Audio*

After stopping the tape player, check the words you have written against the words in the left-hand column. If any words are misspelled, practice writing them correctly. When you feel that you know and understand the words, go on to the Terminology Practice.

PRACTICE

____

____

____

____

____

Name ______________________ Date ______________ Errors ________

LESSON 67: TERMINOLOGY PRACTICE

Drugs: Integumentary and Genitourinary Systems

Without looking at your previous work, write the word that is described by each definition. Since many of the drugs in this section have similar uses, the first letter of the drug matching the definition is given.

DEFINITION	TERM
1. Brand name for the generic drug nitrofurantoin macrocrystals, prescribed as an antibacterial agent in urinary tract infections	M ______________
2. Brand name for clotrimazole, prescribed as an antifungal agent in skin infections	L ______________
3. Brand name for the generic drug betamethasone dipropionate, prescribed to relieve inflammation, itching and swelling of the skin	D ______________
4. Brand name for the generic drug sulfisoxazole, which is prescribed for the treatment of infections of the urinary tract	A ______________
5. The generic name of a drug prescribed for several skin problems characterized by itching, swelling, redness, etc.	h ______________
6. Brand name for oxybutynin chloride, which is prescribed for the relief of symptoms of urinary instability	D ______________
7. Brand name for the generic drug isotretinoin, prescribed for patients with severe acne	A ______________
8. Brand name for bethanechol chloride, used for the treatment of postoperative and postpartum nonobstructive urinary retention	U ______________
9. Brand name for the generic drug tretinoin, used in the treatment of some kinds of acne	R ______________
10. Brand name for the generic drug acyclovir, used in the treatment of genital herpes	Z ______________
11. Brand name of the generic drug trimethoprim sulfamethoxazole, used in the treatment of types of urinary tract infections	S ______________
12. Brand name for the generic drug lindane, used for the treatment of scabies	K ______________
13. Brand name for the generic drug nystatin and neomycin sulfate, used for the control of dermatitis	M ______________

14. Brand name for the generic drug phenozopyridine hydrochloride, prescribed for the relief of urinary pain, urgency, frequency, etc. P ____________________

15. The brand name of the generic drug ciprofloxacin, an antibacterial agent used to treat a variety of infections C ____________________

Check your answers against the word and definition lists on the first page of this lesson. If you have any errors, count them and write the number in the blank at the top of the page. Practice any missed or misspelled words in the space provided. Sign your work and give it to your instructor. You are now ready for the next lesson.

PRACTICE

LESSON

68

Terminology Presentation

Drugs: Nervous and Respiratory Systems

Listen to the Lab Tape provided by your instructor, and you will hear the words presented in this lesson. Read the words as they are said, noticing spelling and pronunciation. The recording will tell you when the presentation for this lesson is completed and will give you any further instructions. Do not go on to the next recorded lesson until you have completed Lesson 68 and feel that you know the words that have been presented.

• • • ▶ *Start Audio*

WORD	DEFINITION	ANSWER
1. Tegretol (Teg′rit-tahl)	Brand name for carbamazepine, used to control epilepsy and also the pain from trigeminal neuralgia	1. ________
2. Proventil (Pro-ven′til)	Brand name for the generic drug albuterol, prescribed for the relief of breathing difficulty	2. ________
3. phenobarbital (fen-o-bar′bi-tahl)	The generic name for various brand name drugs prescribed as a sleep-producing agent and sedative	3. ________
4. Cogentin (Ko-jen′tin)	Brand name for benztropine mesylate, prescribed to control abnormal movements and muscle stiffness associated with Parkinson's disease	4. ________
5. Phenergan (Fen′er-gan)	Brand name for promethazine hydrochloride alcohol, a syrup prescribed for the relief of nasal and chest congestion	5. ________
6. Organidin (Or-gan′i-din)	Brand name for iodinated glycerol, prescribed as an expectorant in respiratory conditions such as bronchitis	6. ________
7. Valium (Val′e-um)	Brand name for diazepam, used for the relief of anxiety and tension	7. ________
8. penicillin (pen-i-sil′in)	Ampicillin. The generic name for a variety of brand names such as V-cillin K, Ledercillin VK and PenVee K, used to treat a variety of infections	8. ________

9. Dilantin (Di-lan′tin)	Brand name for diphenylhydantoin sodium, used in the treatment of patients suffering from convulsive disorders such as epilepsy	9. ________
10. Sinemet (Sin′e-met)	Brand name for levodopa, which is prescribed for the treatment of patients with Parkinson's disease	10. ________
11. Theo-Dur (The-o-dur′)	Brand name for theophylline, which is used in the treatment of patients suffering from respiratory diseases such as asthma, bronchitis and emphysema	11. ________
12. codeine (ko′den)	Generic name for a variety of brand name drugs used as an antitussive and analgesic agent	12. ________
13. Halcion (Hal-se′on)	Brand name for triazolam, used as an agent to treat insomnia as well as for the relief of anxiety and tension	13. ________
14. Alupent (Al′u-pent)	Brand name for metaproterenol sulfate, used in the treatment of breathing difficulties in patients with asthma, bronchitis and emphysema	14. ________
15. epinephrine (ep′e-nef′rin)	Generic name of a drug used to treat bronchial asthma, some allergic disorders, glaucoma and heart block; also used as a topical and local vasoconstrictor	15. ________

■ • • • *Stop Audio at Tone*

Study the 15 words for this lesson. Practice each word several times on a separate sheet of paper, checking your spelling and repeating the meaning to yourself. Listen to the recording and pronounce the words as many times as necessary. When you feel that you know the words well, you are ready to go on to the next step.

Use a sheet of paper to cover all columns except the Answer Column on the previous page. The words you have learned will be presented again on the recording. As each word is pronounced, write it in the space provided in the Answer Column.

• • • ▶ *Start Audio*

After stopping the tape player, check the words you have written against the words in the left-hand column. If any words are misspelled, practice writing them correctly. When you feel that you know and understand the words, go on to the Terminology Practice.

Name ______________________________ Date ____________________ Errors __________

LESSON 68: TERMINOLOGY PRACTICE

Drugs: Nervous and Respiratory Systems

Without looking at your previous work, write the word that is described by each definition. Since many of the drugs in this section have similar uses, the first letter of the drug matching the definition is given.

DEFINITION	TERM
1. Brand name for triazolam, used as an agent to treat insomnia as well as for the relief of anxiety and tension	H ____________________
2. Brand name for diphenylhydantoin sodium, used in the treatment of patients suffering from convulsive disorders such as epilepsy	D ____________________
3. Brand name for iodinated glycerol, prescribed as an expectorant in respiratory conditions such as bronchitis	O ____________________
4. Brand name of theophylline, which is used in the treatment of patients suffering from respiratory diseases such as asthma, bronchitis and emphysema	T ____________________
5. Generic name of a drug used to treat bronchial asthma, some allergic disorders, glaucoma and heart block; also as a topical and local vasoconstrictor	e ____________________
6. The generic name for various brand name drugs prescribed as a sleep-producing agent and sedative	p ____________________
7. Generic name for a variety of brand name drugs used as an antitussive and analgesic agent	c ____________________
8. Brand name for metaproterenol sulfate, used in the treatment of breathing difficulties in patients with asthma, bronchitis and emphysema	A ____________________
9. Brand name for diazepam, used for the relief of anxiety and tension	V ____________________
10. Brand name for the generic drug albuterol, prescribed for the relief of breathing difficulty	P ____________________
11. Brand name for promethazine hydrochloride alcohol, a syrup prescribed for the relief of nasal and chest congestion	P ____________________
12. Brand name for levodopa, which is prescribed for the treatment of patients with Parkinson's disease	S ____________________

13. The generic name for a variety of brand names such as V-cillin K, Ledercillin VK and PenVee K, used to treat a variety of infections p ____________________

14. Brand name for carbamazepine, used to control epilepsy and also the pain from trigeminal neuralgia T____________________

15. Brand name for benztropine mesylate, prescribed to control abnormal movements and muscle stiffness associated with Parkinson's disease C____________________

Check your answers against the word and definition lists on the first page of this lesson. If you have any errors, count them and write the number in the blank at the top of the page. Practice any missed or misspelled words in the space provided. Sign your work and give it to your instructor. You are now ready for the next lesson.

PRACTICE

LESSON

69

Terminology Presentation

Drugs: Digestive System and Organs of Special Sense

Listen to the Lab Tape provided by your instructor, and you will hear the words presented in this lesson. Read the words as they are said, noticing spelling and pronunciation. The recording will tell you when the presentation for this lesson is completed and will give you any further instructions. Do not go on to the next recorded lesson until you have completed Lesson 69 and feel that you know the words that have been presented.

• • • ▸ *Start Audio*

WORD	DEFINITION	ANSWER
1. Bentyl (Ben′til)	Brand name for dicyclomine hydrochloride, used in the treatment of peptic ulcer and other gastrointestinal disorders	1. ________
2. Diamox (Di′a-moks)	Brand name for the generic drug acetazolamide, an enzyme inhibitor used to treat edema, epilepsy and glaucoma	2. ________
3. Timoptic (Tim-op′tik)	Brand name for timolol maleate, prescribed for the treatment of glaucoma. It lowers elevated eye pressure	3. ________
4. Zantac (Zan′tak)	Brand name for the generic drug ranitidine hydrochloride, used for the treatment of patients with duodenal and gastric ulcers	4. ________
5. Tagamet (Tag′ah-met)	Brand name for cimetidine, prescribed to lower acid secretion in the stomach; indicated in the treatment of duodenal ulcers	5. ________
6. Neosporin (Ne-o-spor′in) ophthalmic solution	Brand name for polymyxin B-neomycin indicated for the short term treatment of eye infections	6. ________
7. Naphcon A (Naf′kon A)	Eye drop solution used in the treatment of eye irritation or allergic or inflammatory eye problems	7. ________
8. Lomotil (Lo-mo′til)	Brand name for atropine sulfate, prescribed for the treatment of diarrhea	8. ________
9. Axid (Ake′sid)	Brand name for nizatidine, used for the treatment of duodenal ulcer	9. ________

10. Ilotycin (I-lo-ti′sin)	Brand name for erythromycin, indicated in the treatment of various infections. Ilotycin eye ointment is used in the treatment of eye infections	**10.** ____________
11. Propine (Pro′pin)	Brand name for dipivefrin hydrochloride, used to control internal eye pressure in glaucoma	**11.** ____________
12. Reglan (Reg′lan)	Brand name for metoclopramide hydrochloride, prescribed for the relief of gastrointestinal symptoms in some diabetic patients	**12.** ____________
13. Beconase (Be′ko-naz)	Brand name for beclomethasone dipropionate indicated for the relief of symptoms of rhinitis	**13.** ____________
14. Colace (Ko′las)	Brand name for docusate sodium, used to keep stools soft for easy, natural passage	**14.** ____________
15. Imodium (I-mod′e-um)	Brand name for loperamide hydrochloride, used in the treatment of diarrhea	**15.** ____________

■ • • • *Stop Audio at Tone*

Study the 15 words for this lesson. Practice each word several times, checking your spelling and repeating the meaning to yourself. Listen to the recording and pronounce the words as many times as necessary. When you feel that you know the words well, you are ready to go on to the next step.

Use a sheet of paper to cover all columns except the Answer Column on the previous page. The words you have learned will be presented again on the recording. As each word is pronounced, write it in the space provided in the Answer Column.

• • • ▸ *Start Audio*

After stopping the tape player, check the words you have written against the words in the left-hand column. If any words are misspelled, practice writing them correctly. When you feel that you know and understand the words, go on to the Terminology Practice.

PRACTICE

____

____

____

____

____

Name ______________________________ Date ____________________ Errors __________

LESSON 69: TERMINOLOGY PRACTICE

Drugs: Digestive System and Organs of Special Sense

Without looking at your previous work, write the word that is described by each definition. Since many of the drugs in this section have similar uses, the first letter of the drug matching the definition is given.

DEFINITION	TERM
1. Brand name for the generic drug ranitidine hydrochloride, used for the treatment of patients with duodenal and gastric ulcers	Z__________
2. Brand name for dipivefrin hydrochloride, used to control internal eye pressure in glaucoma	P __________
3. Brand name for loperamide hydrochloride, used in the treatment of diarrhea	I __________
4. Brand name for the generic drug acetazolamide, an enzyme inhibitor used to treat edema, epilepsy and glaucoma	D__________
5. Brand name for metoclopramide hydrochloride, prescribed for the relief of gastrointestinal symptoms in some diabetic patients	R__________
6. Brand name for dicyclomine hydrochloride, used in the treatment of peptic ulcer and other gastrointestinal disorders	B __________
7. Brand name for docusate sodium, used to keep stools soft for easy, natural passage	C__________
8. Brand name for beclomethasone dipropionate, indicated for the relief of symptoms of rhinitis	B __________
9. Brand name for cimetidine, prescribed to lower acid secretion in the stomach; indicated in the treatment of duodenal ulcers	T __________
10. Eye drop solution used in the treatment of eye irritation or allergic or inflammatory eye problems	N__________
11. Brand name for polymyxin B-neomycin indicated for the short term treatment of eye infections	N__________
12. Brand name for erythromycin, indicated in the treatment of various infections. The eye ointment is used in the treatment of eye infections	I __________

13. Brand name for atropine sulfate, prescribed for the treatment of diarrhea — L__________________

14. Brand name for timolol maleate, prescribed for the treatment of glaucoma. It lowers elevated eye pressure — T__________________

15. Brand name for nizatidine, used for the treatment of duodenal ulcer — A__________________

Check your answers against the word and definition lists on the first page of this lesson. If you have any errors, count them and write the number in the blank at the top of the page. Practice any missed or misspelled words in the space provided. Sign your work and give it to your instructor. You are now ready for the next lesson.

PRACTICE

LESSON

70

Terminology Presentation

Drugs: Endocrine, Hemic and Lymphatic Systems

Listen to the Lab Tape provided by your instructor, and you will hear the words presented in this lesson. Read the words as they are said, noticing spelling and pronunciation. The recording will tell you when the presentation for this lesson is completed and will give you any further instructions. Do not go on to the next recorded lesson until you have completed Lesson 70 and feel that you know the words that have been presented.

• • • ▶ *Start Audio*

WORD	DEFINITION	ANSWER
1. Lupron (Lu'pron)	Brand name for leuprolide acetate, prescribed for the palliative treatment of prostatic cancer	1. ________
2. heparin (hep'ah-rin)	Generic name of a drug indicated for anticoagulant therapy	2. ________
3. Trental (Tren'tal)	Brand name for pentoxifylline, used to increase blood flow in patients with muscle pain	3. ________
4. Glucotrol (Glu'ka-trol)	Brand name for glipizide, given to control blood sugar levels in diabetics	4. ________
5. Cytoxan (Si-taks'an)	Brand name for cyclophosphamide, indicated in the treatment of several types of malignant neoplastic diseases	5. ________
6. Synthroid (Sin'throid)	Brand name for levothyroxine sodium, prescribed for patients who have a decreased amount of thyroid hormone production	6. ________
7. Compazine (Komp'ah-zen)	Brand name for prochlorperazine maleate, used for the treatment of certain psychotic disorders	7. ________
8. Nolvadex (Nol'va-deks)	Brand name for tamoxifen citrate, used for the treatment of female breast cancer	8. ________
9. Persantine (Per-san'ten)	Brand name for dipyridamole, indicated to increase the blood flow following surgical cardiac valve replacement	9. ________

10. DiaBeta (Di-ah-bet'a)	Brand name for glyburide, used to control blood sugar levels in diabetic patients	**10.** ________________
11. Demulen (Dem'u-len)	Brand name for ethynodiol diacetate, used as an oral contraceptive	**11.** ________________
12. Premarin (Prem'a-rin)	Brand name for conjugated estrogens, generally prescribed as estrogenic replacement therapy	**12.** ________________
13. Coumadin (Ku'ma-din)	Brand name for crystalline sodium warfarin, used for the prevention of blood clots	**13.** ________________
14. Tigan (Ti'gan)	Brand name for trimethobenzamide hydrochloride, prescribed to control nausea and vomiting	**14.** ________________
15. Micronase (Mi-kro-nas')	Brand name for glyburide, used to control blood sugar levels in diabetic patients	**15.** ________________

■ • • • *Stop Audio at Tone*

Study the 15 words for this lesson. Practice each word several times, checking your spelling and repeating the meaning to yourself. Listen to the recording and pronounce the words as many times as necessary. When you feel that you know the words well, you are ready to go on to the next step.

Use a sheet of paper to cover all columns except the Answer Column on the previous page. The words you have learned will be presented again on the recording. As each word is pronounced, write it in the space provided in the Answer Column.

• • • ▶ *Start Audio*

After stopping the tape player, check the words you have written against the words in the left-hand column. If any words are misspelled, practice writing them correctly. When you feel that you know and understand the words, go on to the Terminology Practice.

PRACTICE

____

____

____

____

____

____

____

Name ______________________________ Date ____________________ Errors __________

LESSON 70: TERMINOLOGY PRACTICE

Drugs: Endocrine, Hemic and Lymphatic Systems

Without looking at your previous work, write the word that is described by each definition. Since many of the drugs in this section have similar uses, the first letter of the drug matching the definition is given.

DEFINITION	TERM
1. Brand name for glyburide, used to control blood sugar levels in diabetic patients	D ____________
2. Brand name for tamoxifen citrate, used for the treatment of female breast cancer	N ____________
3. Brand name for levothyroxine sodium, prescribed for patients who have a decreased amount of thyroid hormone production	S ____________
4. Brand name for trimethobenzamide hydrochloride, prescribed to control nausea and vomiting	T ____________
5. Brand name for ethynodiol diacetate, used as an oral contraceptive	D ____________
6. Brand name for pentoxifylline, used to increase blood flow in patients with muscle pain	T ____________
7. Brand name for conjugated estrogens, generally prescribed as estrogen replacement therapy	P ____________
8. Brand name for leuprolide acetate, prescribed for the palliative treatment of prostatic cancer	L ____________
9. Brand name for crystalline sodium warfarin, used for the prevention of blood clots	C ____________
10. Brand name for cyclophosphamide, indicated in the treatment of several types of malignant neoplastic diseases	C ____________
11. Brand name for prochlorperazine maleate, used for the treatment of certain psychotic disorders	C ____________
12. Generic name of a drug indicated for anticoagulant therapy	h ____________
13. Brand name for dipyridamole, indicated to increase the blood flow following surgical valve replacement	P ____________

14. Brand name for glipizide, given to control blood sugar levels in diabetics G ______________________

15. Brand name for glyburide, used to control blood sugar levels in diabetic patients M______________________

Check your answers against the word and definition lists on the first page of this lesson. If you have any errors, count them and write the number in the blank at the top of the page. Practice any missed or misspelled words in the space provided. Sign your work and give it to your instructor. You are now ready for the next lesson.

PRACTICE

Name ________________________ Date ______________ Errors ________

LESSON 71 TERMINOLOGY REVIEW FOR TEST 14

This is a review of the words you have learned in the preceding five lessons.

Unlike the review for Test 13, the words are not written out for you. As each word is pronounced on the Lab Tape, write it in the appropriate numbered blank on the left, then write the appropriate definition in the space to the right.

• • • ▸ *Start Audio*

WORD	MEANING OR DEFINITION
1. ____________	____________
2. ____________	____________
3. ____________	____________
4. ____________	____________
5. ____________	____________
6. ____________	____________
7. ____________	____________
8. ____________	____________

9. ______________________ ______________________________

10. ______________________ ______________________________

11. ______________________ ______________________________

12. ______________________ ______________________________

13. ______________________ ______________________________

14. ______________________ ______________________________

15. ______________________ ______________________________

■ • • • *Stop Audio at Tone*

After all 15 words have been written, write the definition of each one. Use the Glossary or a medical dictionary to check your spellings and definitions. Practice the words on a separate sheet of paper, paying particular attention to any you missed or misspelled.

When you feel you know the words and definitions well, sign your work, indicate the number of errors, and turn your work in to your instructor. You are now ready for the Extra Credit Review (if your instructor assigns it) or Test 14.

Name ______________________ Date ______________ Errors ________

LESSON 71 | EXTRA CREDIT REVIEW

This Extra Credit Review should be done at the discretion of your instructor. If you are instructed to complete this portion of the Review, turn it in to your instructor when you are finished.

PART A

Write the definition of the following 20 drugs to the right of the given drug.

TERM	DEFINITION
1. Glucotrol	______________________
2. Plaquenil	______________________
3. Valium	______________________
4. Codeine	______________________
5. Mycolog	______________________
6. Timoptic	______________________
7. Compazine	______________________
8. quinidine	______________________
9. phenobarbital	______________________
10. penicillin	______________________
11. Azo Gantrisin	______________________
12. Diamox	______________________
13. Axid	______________________
14. DiaBeta	______________________
15. Tigan	______________________
16. Alupent	______________________
17. Cipro	______________________
18. Naphcon A	______________________
19. Premarin	______________________
20. Zantac	______________________

PART B

Match the following definitions with the drug given. Place the correct letter of the definition given to the left of the drug name.

TERM

_____ 21. Tagamet

_____ 22. Imodium

_____ 23. Cytoxan

_____ 24. Kwell

_____ 25. Premarin

_____ 26. Phenergan

_____ 27. epinephrine

_____ 28. captopril

_____ 29. Prednisone

_____ 30. Septra

DEFINITION

a. Generic name of a drug used to treat bronchial asthma, some allergic disorders, glaucoma and heart block; also as a topical and local vasoconstrictor
b. Generic name for Capoten, a drug prescribed for high blood pressure in patients who have normal kidney function
c. Brand name for loperamide hydrochloride, used in the treatment of diarrhea
d. The generic name of a drug prescribed as an antiinflammatory agent
e. Brand name for cimetidine, prescribed to lower acid secretion in the stomach; indicated in the treatment of duodenal ulcers
f. Brand name for conjugated estrogens, generally prescribed as estrogen replacement therapy
g. Brand name for promethazine hydrochloride alcohol, a syrup prescribed for the relief of nasal and chest congestion
h. Brand name for the generic drug lindane, used for the treatment of scabies
i. Brand name of the generic drug trimethoprim sulfamethoxazole, used in the treatment of types of urinary tract infections
j. Brand name for cyclophosphamide, indicated in the treatment of several types of malignant neoplastic diseases

You may now go on to Test 14.

Glossary

A

Aboral	Situated away from or remote from the mouth.
Abrasion	The wearing away or wearing down of the teeth.
Abutment	Tooth that provides the point of anchorage for a bridge.
Accutane	Brand name for the generic drug isotretinoin, prescribed for patients with severe acne.
Acrylic resins	Plastic materials used in the fabrication of bridges and crowns.
Adduct	To draw toward.
Aden(o)	A word element denoting the glands.
Adenemphraxis	Glandular obstruction.
Adenitis	Inflammation of a gland.
Adenoblast	An embryonic cell producing glandular tissue.
Adenocarcinoma	Glandular cancer or carcinoma.
Adenodynia	Gland pain.
Adenohypersthenia	Excessive glandular activity.
Adenoid	Like or resembling a gland.
Adenoma	A benign tumor of a gland.
Adren(o)	Pertaining to the adrenal glands.
Adrenalectomy	Surgical removal of the adrenal gland.
Adrenalinuria	Presence of epinephrine in the urine.
Adrenalitis	Inflammation of the adrenal gland.
Adrenokinetic	Stimulating the adrenal gland.
Adrenomegaly	Enlargement of the adrenal gland.
Adrenopathy	Any disease of the adrenal gland.
Adrenoprival	Pertaining to loss or deprivation of the adrenal gland.
Adrenotoxin	Toxic or poisonous to the adrenal gland.
Albuminuria	Presence of serum albumin in the urine.
Aldactazide	Brand name for the drug spironolactone, used to treat high blood pressure and water accumulation in body tissue.
Algesia	A word element, usually a suffix, denoting pain or ache.
Algia	A word element denoting pain or ache.

Allergist (Allergy)	A specialist concerned with the diagnosis and treatment of allergies.
Allopurinol	The generic name for Zyloprim, prescribed for the treatment of gout.
Alloy	The product formed as a result of combining two or more metals.
Alupent	Brand name for metaproterenol sulfate, used in the treatment of breathing difficulties in patients with asthma, bronchitis and emphysema.
Amalgam	An alloy used to fill teeth containing mercury, silver and tin.
Amaurosis	Blindness.
Ambilateral	Pertaining to both the right and left side.
Amblyopia	Lazy or dull eye.
Analgesic	Pertaining to the giving of a medicine to relieve pain.
Anastomosis	An opening or connection between two vessels or organs.
Anemia	Reduction of the number of red blood cells in the blood.
Anesthesiologist (Anesthesiology)	Specialist who studies and administers anesthetic agents.
Angi(o)	Word element denoting vessels.
Angiectasis	Dilatation of a blood vessel.
Angiogram	X-ray picture of a blood vessel.
Angiomegaly	Enlarged blood vessel.
Angiomyolipoma	Tumor of blood vessels, muscle, and fat.
Angiospasm	Contraction of a blood vessel.
Angiostenosis	Narrowing of the lumen of a blood vessel.
Angiostomy	Making an opening into a blood vessel.
Ankyloglossia	Tongue-tied.
Anterosuperior	Situated above and in front of something.
Antiemetic	An agent that prevents nausea and vomiting.
Apnea	Temporary absence of breathing.
Apobiosis	Not living.
Appliance	A device worn by a dental patient during the course of treatment.
Art, arteri(o)	Pertaining to the arteries.
Arterial	Of or pertaining to the arteries.
Arteriectasis	Dilatation of an artery.
Arteriopathy	A disease of an artery.
Arteriorrhaphy	Suture of an artery.
Arteriorrhexis	Rupture of an artery.
Arteriosclerosis	Hardening of the walls of an artery.
Arteriostrepsis	Twisting of an artery to stop bleeding.
Arteritis	Inflammation of an artery.
Arthr(o)	Word element denoting the joints.
Arthralgia	Pain in a joint.
Arthritis	Inflammation of a joint.

Arthrocentesis	Surgical puncture of a joint.
Arthrodesis	Operative fixation of a joint dislocation using the joint ligaments.
Arthrodysplasia	Abnormal joint development.
Arthrolith	A calcium deposit in a joint.
Arthropathy	Any disease affecting a joint.
Arthrophyma	Swelling of a joint.
Arthroscope	An endoscope for examination of the interior of a joint.
Arthrosynovitis	Inflammation of the synovial membrane of a joint.
Articulate	To unite the teeth of one arch in the proper position with the teeth of the opposing arch.
Articulator	An instrument for holding the casts of the jaws or teeth in the proper relationship to one another.
Attrition	The wearing away of teeth.
Axid	Brand name for nizatidine, used for the treatment of duodenal ulcer.
Azo Gantrisin	Brand name for the generic drug sulfisoxazole, which is prescribed for the treatment of infections of the urinary tract.

B

Bacterial plaque	A film-like covering of the teeth.
Bacteriuria	Presence of bacteria in the urine.
Baseplate	A sheet of wax or metal that is used for trial denture setups.
Basophil	A cell or structure staining readily with basic dyes.
Beconase	Brand name for beclomethasone dipropionate, indicated for the relief of symptoms of rhinitis.
Bentyl	Brand name for dicyclomine hydrochloride, used in the treatment of peptic ulcer and other gastrointestinal disorders.
Biceps	A muscle having two heads.
Bicuspids	Teeth with two cusps, situated between cuspids and molars.
Blephar(o)	Word element denoting the eyelid.
Blepharitis	Inflammation of the eyelid.
Blepharodiastasis	Excessive separation of the eyelids, causing the eyes to open very wide.
Blepharoplasty	Plastic surgery on the eyelid.
Blepharoptosis	Drooping of the eyelid.
Blepharorrhaphy	Surgical repair of the eyelid.
Blepharosynechia	The growing together or adhesions of the eyelid.
Bradycardia	Abnormally slow heartbeat.
Bronch(o)	A word part denoting the bronchi (plural) or bronchus (singular), the air passages within the lungs.
Bronchiectasis	Dilatation of the bronchi.
Bronchitis	Inflammation of the bronchi.
Bronchoedema	Swelling of the mucosa of the bronchi.
Bronchoplegia	Paralysis of the bronchi.

Bronchopneumonitis	Inflammation of the lungs originating at the bronchi.
Bronchorrhea	Excessive secretion of mucus from the bronchial mucous membrane.
Bronchoscopy	Inspection or examination of the bronchi.
Bruxism	The clenching or grinding of the teeth.
Burnishing	Polishing by friction.

C

Captopril	Generic name for Capoten, a drug prescribed for high blood pressure in patients who have normal kidney function.
Cardi(o), cardi(a)	Word element denoting the heart.
Cardiac	Of or pertaining to the heart.
Cardiogram	The recording of the heart's movements.
Cardiograph	An instrument for recording the heart rate.
Cardiologist (Cardiology)	Specialist in the diagnosis and treatment of heart disorders.
Cardiomegaly	Enlargement of the heart.
Cardiopathy	A disease of the heart.
Cardiorrhaphy	Suture of surgical repair of the heart.
Cardiospasm	A contraction of the heart.
Cardiotomy	Surgical incision into the heart.
Carditis	Inflammation of the heart.
Caries	Decay of tooth structure.
Cataphasia	A speech disorder in which the same word or phrase is constantly repeated.
Centimeter	A unit of the metric system being one hundredth part of a meter.
Cephal(o)	A word part denoting the head.
Cephaledema	Swelling or edema of the head.
Cephalic	Pertaining to the head.
Cephalocaudal	Pertaining to the long axis of the body (head to tail).
Cephalocele	Hernial protrusion of part of the cranial contents.
Cephalocentesis	Surgical puncture of the skull or head to draw off fluid.
Cephalometer	Instrument to measure the head.
Cephaloplegia	Paralysis of the head muscle.
Cheil(o)	A combining form denoting the lip.
Cheilectomy	Excision of the lip as for cheilocarcinoma.
Cheilitis	Inflammation of the lip.
Cheilocarcinoma	Cancer of the lip.
Cheilophagia	Habit of biting the lip.
Cheilorrhaphy	Suture of the lip.
Cheiloschisis	Cleft in the lip; harelip.
Cheilostomatoplasty	Plastic surgery on the lip and mouth.

Cheilotomy	Incision into the lip.
Cheir(o)	A word element denoting the hands.
Cheirarthritis	Inflammation of the joints of the hands.
Cheirobrachialgia	Painful condition of the hand and arm.
Cheiromegaly	Enlargement of the hands.
Cheiroplasty	Plastic surgery on the hand.
Cheiropodalgia	Pain in the hands and feet.
Cheirospasm	Contraction of the hand.
Chest specialist (Pulmonary disease)	Specialist in the diagnosis and treatment of diseases of the chest.
Chir(o)	A word element denoting the hands.
Chiropractic	A system of therapeutics which attempts to restore normal function of the body by manipulation of the human body.
Chlorophyll	The green coloring matter of plants.
Cholecyst(o)	A word element denoting the gall bladder.
Cholecystectomy	Excision of the gall bladder.
Cholecystitis	Inflammation of the gall bladder.
Cholecystography	X-ray examination of the gall bladder.
Cholecystoptosis	Downward displacement of the gall bladder.
Choledoch(o)	Word element denoting the common bile duct.
Choledochogastrostomy	Surgical connection between the stomach and bile duct.
Choledocholithotripsy	Crushing of a stone in the common bile duct.
Choledochotomy	Incision into the common bile duct.
Cholelithiasis	Gall stones.
Chondr(o)	Word element denoting cartilage.
Chondritis	Inflammation of the cartilage.
Chondrocostal	Pertaining to the ribs and cartilages.
Chondrodysplasia	Abnormal formation of cartilage.
Chondrolipoma	A cartilaginous and fatty tissue tumor.
Chondrolysis	Degeneration of cartilage.
Chondropathy	Any disease of cartilage.
Chondrophyte	A cartilaginous growth at the articular end of a bone.
Chyluria	Presence of chyle in the urine.
Cipro	The brand name of the generic drug ciprofloxacin, an antibacterial agent used to treat a variety of infections.
Cirrhosis	A liver disorder in which the primary symptom is jaundice.
Codeine	Generic name for a variety of brand name drugs used as an antitussive and analgesic agent.
Cogentin	Brand name for benztropine mesylate, prescribed to control abnormal movements and muscle stiffness associated with Parkinson's disease.
Colace	Brand name for docusate sodium, used to keep stools soft for easy natural passage.

Compazine	Brand name for prochlorperazine maleate, used for the treatment of certain psychotic disorders.
Contact point	The area of a tooth's surface that touches a neighboring tooth.
Contraindication	Any condition which renders a certain treatment undesirable.
Costalgia	Rib pain.
Coumadin	Brand name for crystalline sodium warfarin, used for the prevention of blood clots.
Crani(o)	Word element denoting the skull or cranium.
Craniectomy	Surgical removal of part of the skull.
Craniocele	A protrusion of a part of the cranial contents through a defect in the skull.
Craniomalacia	Softening of the skull.
Cranioplasty	Plastic surgery on the cranium.
Craniorachischisis	Congenital fissure of the skull and spinal column.
Craniospinal	Pertaining to the skull and spine.
Craniotomy	Incision into the skull.
Crown	The part of a tooth that is covered with enamel and projects from the gum.
Crown and bridge	The branch of dentistry concerned with the replacement of natural tooth structures with dental prostheses.
Crymodynia	Rheumatic pain coming on in cold or damp weather.
Cryptorchidism	A congenital failure of the testes to descend into the scrotum.
Cuspid	A tooth with a point or cusp.
Cyanemia	Bluishness of the blood.
Cyt(o)	A word element denoting cells.
Cytobiology	The biology of cells.
Cytodiagnosis	Diagnosis of disease by the use of cells.
Cytolysis	Destruction or dissolution of cells.
Cytoma	A cell tumor.
Cytometaplasia	Change in the form or function of a cell.
Cytomorphology	Study of the shape of cells.
Cytotoxicity	Being poisonous or toxic to cells.
Cytoxan	Brand name for cyclophosphamide, indicated in the treatment of several types of malignant neoplastic diseases.

D

Dacry(o)	A word part denoting tears or the lacrimal (tear) glands or ducts.
Dacryoadenitis	Inflammation of the lacrimal or tear gland.
Dacryocyst	A lacrimal or tear sac.
Dacryocystitis	Inflammation of the tear sac.
Dacryolithiasis	A stone or concretion in a lacrymal gland or duct.
Dacryoma	A tumor of the lacrimal apparatus.

Dacryorrhea	Excessive discharge of tears.
Dacryostenosis	Narrowing of the lacrymal duct.
Decagram	Ten grams.
Deciliter	One tenth of a liter.
Dehydrate	To remove water from a substance such as the body.
Demilune	Half moon or crescent shaped.
Demulen	Brand name for ethynodiol diacetate, used as an oral contraceptive.
Dental arch	The curved structure of natural dentition.
Dental hygienist	A person trained in the art of dental prophylaxis.
Dental technician	A person trained in the fabrication of dental appliances or devices (dentures, etc.).
Dentin	The tissue that constitutes the chief substance of a tooth.
Denture	An artificial substitute for natural teeth.
Derm(a), derm(o), dermat(o)	A word element denoting the skin.
Dermal	Of or pertaining to the skin.
Dermalgia	Skin pain.
Dermatitis	Inflammation of the skin.
Dermatoautoplasty	Autografting of skin taken from another part of the patient's own body.
Dermatoconiosis	An occupational dermatitis caused by irritation by dust.
Dermatologist (Dermatology)	Specialist in the diagnosis and treatment of skin disorders.
Dermatome	An instrument for cutting the skin or thin skin grafts.
Dermatophobia	A morbid fear of acquiring a skin disease.
Dermatorrhea	An excessive secretion of the sebaceous or sweat glands of the skin.
Dermatosis	Any generalized skin disease.
Dermomycosis	Any fungus disease of the skin.
DiaBeta	Brand name for glyburide, used to control blood sugar levels in diabetic patients.
Diamox	Brand name for the generic drug acetazolamide, an enzyme inhibitor used to treat edema, epilepsy and glaucoma.
Digoxin	The generic name of a drug which increases the contractions of the heart.
Dilantin	Brand name for diphenylhydantoin sodium, used in the treatment of patients suffering from convulsive disorders such as epilepsy.
Diplophonia	The product of double voice sounds.
Diprolene	Brand name for the generic drug betamethasone dipropionate, prescribed to relieve inflammation, itching and swelling of the skin.
Dips(ia), dips(o)	A word element denoting thirst.
Dipsogen	A condition producing thirst.
Dipsomania	A compulsion or uncontrolled desire to drink spiritous liquor.

Dipsosis	A condition producing thirst.
Dipsotherapy	Treatment by limitation of water ingested.
Ditropan	Brand name for oxybutynin chloride, which is prescribed for the relief of symptoms of urinary instability.
Dorsal	Pertaining to the back.
Dyskinesia	Difficult or painful movement.
Dyspnea	Difficult breathing.
Dysuria	Painful or difficult urination.

E

Ectoderm	The outermost layers of skin.
Edentulous	Without teeth.
Emia	A word element denoting relationship to the blood.
Enamel	The hard tissue that covers the dentin of the crown part of a tooth.
Encephal(o)	A word part denoting the brain.
Encephalitis	Inflammation of the brain.
Encephalodysplasia	Any congenital abnormality of the brain.
Encephalogram	X-ray picture of the brain.
Encephaloma	A brain tumor.
Encephalomalacia	Morbid softening of the brain.
Encephalopathic	Pertaining to a brain disease.
Encephalothlipsis	Compression of the brain.
Endocarditis	Inflammation within the heart.
Endocrinologist (Endocrinology)	A specialist who studies the internally secreting glands and their effect on the body and its metabolism.
Endodontics	The branch of dentistry concerned with the extraction or removal of teeth.
Enter(o)	A word part denoting the intestines.
Enterauxe	Enlargement of the intestinal wall.
Enterocleisis	Blockage or closure of the intestine.
Enteroclysis	Injection or introduction of liquid into the intestine.
Enterococcus	A type of intestinal bacteria.
Enterokinesis	Muscular movement of the intestinal canal-peristalsis.
Enterolithiasis	Stones or calculi found in the intestine.
Enterorrhagia	Hemorrhage from the intestine.
Enterorrhexis	Rupture of the intestinal wall.
Eosinophil	Attracted or stainable with a rose-colored stain or dye.
Epidemiologist (Epidemiology)	Specializes in the diagnosis and treatment of diseases capable of being communicated from one host to another.
Epinephrine	Generic name of a drug used to treat bronchial asthma, some allergic disorders, glaucoma and heart block; also as a topical and local vasoconstrictor.

Epiotic	Situated above or upon the ear.
Erotomania	Excessive or morbid inclination to erotic thoughts or behavior.
Erythr(o)	A word element denoting red or red blood cells.
Erythroblast	An immature red cell.
Erythroclasis	Breaking up or splitting of red cells.
Erythrocyte	A red blood cell.
Erythrocytosis	An increase in red cells.
Erythroderma	Abnormal redness of the skin over wide areas of the body.
Erythrodontia	Reddish brown pigmentation of the teeth.
Erythropenia	A deficiency in the number of red blood cells.
Erythropoisis	The manufacturing or forming of red blood cells.
Etiology	Study of the cause of a disease.
Eupnea	Normal breathing.
Exodontics	The branch of dentistry concerned with the extraction of teeth.
Extraction	Surgical removal of a tooth.

F

Family practitioner (Family medicine)	Specializes in the diagnosis and treatment of disorders of all members of the family regardless of age or sex, on a continuing basis.
Fasciotomy	Incision into fibrous tissue.
Flexeril	Brand name for the generic drug cyclobenzaprine, used for the relief of muscle spasms or stiffness.
Fluoridation	The addition of fluoride to a community water supply to control dental caries.
Fluoride, topical	The direct application of fluoride to the teeth.
Frenum, labial	The band of tissue inside the lip.
Frenum, lingual	The band of tissue under the tongue.

G

Galact(o)	A combining form denoting milk.
Galactacrasia	Abnormal composition of mother's milk.
Galactogenous	Production of milk by the mammary glands.
Galactophlysis	A vesicular eruption containing a milky fluid.
Galactophoritis	Inflammation of the milk ducts.
Galactopoiesis	Producing milk.
Galactorrhea	Excessive or spontaneous flow of milk.
Galactostasis	Halting or stoppage of milk production.
Gastralgia	Stomach pain.
Gastroenterologist (Gastroenterology)	A specialist that deals with the diagnosis and treatment of diseases of the stomach and intestines.
Gingiva	The tissue enveloping the tooth sockets (gums).

Glaucoma	Opacity of the crystalline lens of the eye in which the eye shows a gray-green color.
Gloss(ia), gloss(o)	Word parts denoting the tongue.
Glossectomy	Surgical removal of all or part of the tongue.
Glossitis	Inflammation of the tongue.
Glossodynia	Tongue pain.
Glossoncus	Swelling or tumor of the tongue.
Glossorrhaphy	Suture or surgical repair of the tongue.
Glossotrichia	Hairy tongue.
Glucotrol	Brand name for glipizide, given to control blood sugar levels in diabetics.
Gyn(o), gynec(o)	Word parts denoting women or the female sex.
Gynandromorphous	Having both male and female qualities.
Gynecologist (Gynecology)	Specialist in the diagnosis and treatment of disorders of women.
Gynecomastia	Excessive development of the male mammary glands or breasts.
Gynephobia	A morbid fear of women.
Gynopathy	Any disease of women.
Gynoplasty	Plastic surgery on the female organs.

H

Halcion	Brand name for triazolam, used as an agent to treat insomnia as well as for the relief of anxiety and tension.
Hectogram	A unit of mass being 100 grams.
Hemangioma	A benign tumor composed of newly formed blood vessels.
Hemarthrosis	Accumulation of blood in a joint cavity.
Hemat(o), hem(o)	A word element denoting the blood.
Hematemesis	Vomiting of blood.
Hematocrit	The volume percentage of red cells to whole blood (separation of red cells for counting).
Hematologist-Oncologist (Hematology-Oncology)	A hematologist deals with the branch of medicine that treats the blood and blood-forming elements. An oncologist deals with tumors, i.e., cancer.
Hematoscheocele	A accumulation of blood in the scrotum.
Hematuria	Presence of blood in the urine.
Hemianesthesia	A condition denoting anesthesia (lack of feeling) on one side.
Hemolysis	Breaking down or destroying blood cells.
Hemophilia	A disease in which the blood clots slowly (bleeder's disease).
Hemoptysis	Spitting or coughing up blood.
Hemostat	An instrument or medicine for stopping bleeding.
Heparin	Generic name of a drug indicated for anticoagulant therapy.
Hepat(o), hepat(ico)	Word parts denoting the liver.
Hepatatrophy	Atrophy or wasting of the liver.

Hepatic	Of or pertaining to the liver.
Hepaticolithotripsy	The operation of crushing a stone in the hepatic duct.
Hepatitis	Inflammation of the liver.
Hepatomegaly	Enlargement of the liver.
Hepatorenal	Pertaining to the liver and kidney.
Hepatorrhaphy	Suture or surgical repair of the liver.
Hist(o), histi(o)	Word elements denoting tissue.
Histanoxia	Oxygen deprivation of tissue, usually resulting from lack of blood supply.
Histocyte	A tissue cell.
Histokinesis	Movement in the tissues of the body.
Histology	A study of tissue.
Histoneurology	The histology of the nervous system.
Historrhexis	Breaking up of tissue.
Histotoxic	Being poisonous to tissue.
Homogenesis	Reproduction by the same process each generation.
Hydrocortisone	The generic name of a drug prescribed for several skin problems characterized by itching, swelling, redness, etc.
Hydrophilic	Attracts or absorbs water.
Hyperalgesia	Increased sensation to pain.
Hyperglycemia	Increased blood sugar.
Hyperpnea	Increase in depth and rate of breathing.
Hypothyroidism	Deficiency in thyroid secretion.
Hyster(o)	A word part denoting the uterus.
Hysteralgia	Pain in the uterus.
Hysterectomy	The removal of the uterus.
Hysterocleisis	Surgical closure of the os uteri.
Hysterocolposcope	An instrument for inspection of the uterine cavity and vagina.
Hysteropexy	Surgical fixation or fastening of the uterus.
Hysterospasm	A uterine spasm.
Hysterostomatomy	An incision into the mouth of the uterus.
Hysterotracheloplasty	Plastic repair of the cervix uteri.

I

Ibuprofen	The generic name for Rufen or Motrin, prescribed as a pain reliever.
Idiosyncrasy	A habit or quality of body or mind peculiar to any individual.
Ile(o)	A word part denoting the ileum, the third or distal portion of the small intestine.
Ileectomy	Surgical removal or excision of the ileum.
Ileitis	Inflammation of the ileum.
Ileocecal	Pertaining to the ileum and cecum.
Ileoentectrophy	Eversion (outward turning) of the ileum.

Ileoproctostomy	Making a surgical connection or opening between the ileum and rectum.
Ileorrhaphy	Suture or surgical repair of the ileum.
Ileotomy	Incision into the ileum.
Ili(o)	A word part denoting the ilium, the superior portion of the hip bone.
Iliac	Of or pertaining to the ilium.
Iliococcygeal	Pertaining to the ilium and coccyx.
Iliocostal	Pertaining to the ilium and ribs.
Iliolumbar	Pertaining to the ilium and lumbar regions.
Iliometer	An instrument for measuring the ilium.
Iliopelvic	Pertaining to the ilium and pelvis.
Iliosacral	Pertaining to the ilium and sacrum.
Ilotycin	Brand name for erythromycin, indicated in the treatment of various infections. Ilotycin eye ointment is used in the treatment of eye infections.
Immunologist (Immunology)	Deals with the body's resistance to disease.
Imodium	Brand name for loperamide hydrochloride, used in the treatment of diarrhea.
Impacted tooth	A tooth embedded in the soft or bony tissues of the jaw that has not totally or partially come through.
Incisor	A tooth with a cutting edge.
Infectious disease	A disease that is capable of being transmitted from one host to another.
Inframammary	Situated below the breast.
Inlay, dental	A cast restoration carved to replace the missing part of a tooth.
Intercostal	Situated between the ribs.
Internist (Internal Medicine)	Specializes in the diagnosis and treatment of the internal structures of the body.
Intrabuccal	Within the cheek or mouth.
Irid(o)	A combining form denoting a relationship to the iris of the eye.
Iridauxesis	Enlargement or thickening of the iris.
Iridectasis	Dilatation of the iris.
Iridomalacia	Softness of the iris.
Iridoplegia	Paralysis of the iris.
Iridosteresis	Loss or absence of the all or part of the iris.
Iridotomy	Incision into the iris.
Iritis	Inflammation of the iris.

J

Jacket	A crown fabricated of porcelain or metal, often called a "cap."

K

Kerat(o)	A word part denoting the cornea of the eye or horny tissue.
Keratectasia	Protrusion of the cornea.
Keratiasis	The presence of horny warts on the skin.
Keratocele	Herniation of a part of the cornea.
Keratocentesis	Surgical puncture of the cornea.
Keratoderma	A horny skin or covering.
Keratogenous	Producing cells that result in the formation of horny tissue such as fingernails.
Keratohelcosis	Ulceration of the cornea.
Keratoid	Like or resembling a horny skin.
Keratoiritis	Inflammation of the cornea and iris.
Keratoma	A tumor or growth of horny tissue.
Keratomycosis	Any fungus disease of the skin.
Keratoplasty	Plastic surgery on the cornea.
Kilounit	A quantity equaling 1000 units.
Kinesalgia	Pain on motion or movement.
Kleptomania	A compulsion to steal.
Kwell	Brand name for the generic drug lindane, used for the treatment of scabies.

L

Laryng(o)	A word part denoting the larynx (voice box).
Laryngeal	Pertaining to the larynx.
Laryngitis	Inflammation of the larynx.
Laryngocentesis	Surgical puncture of the larynx.
Laryngoplegia	Paralysis of the larynx.
Laryngoscope	Instrument used to examine the larynx.
Laryngospasm	Spasmodic closure of the larynx.
Laryngostenosis	Narrowing of the larynx.
Laryngostomy	The creation of an artificial opening into the larynx.
Leukemia	Excessive number of white blood cells.
Lipemia	Abnormally high concentration of fat in the blood.
Lomotil	Brand name for atropine sulfate, used for the treatment of diarrhea.
Lotrimin	Brand name for clotrimazole, prescribed as an antifungal agent in skin infections.
Lupron	Brand name for leuprolide acetate, prescribed for the palliative treatment of prostatic cancer.
Lymph(o)	A combining form indicating lymph or lymphatic vessels or glands.
Lymphadenitis	Inflammation of the lymph gland.
Lymphangioma	A tumor rich in blood vessels.

Lymphedema	Swelling of subcutaneous tissue due to excess lymph fluid.
Lymphocyte	A white cell which is formed in the lymphatic glands.
Lymphocytopenia	Reduction in number of lymphocytes in the blood.
Lymphopathy	Any disease of the lymphatic system.
Lymphopoiesis	Making or developing lymph.
Lymphostasis	Stoppage of lymph flow.

M

Macrodantin	Brand name for the generic drug nitrofurantoin macrocrystals, prescribed as an antibacterial agent in urinary tract infections.
Malar	Referring to the cheek or cheekbone.
Malocclusion	A deviation of normal contact of the upper and lower jaw.
Mandible	The lower jawbone.
Mania, manic	A word ending (suffix) denoting an abnormal love for or compulsion.
Mast(o)	A combining form denoting relationship to the breast or mammary gland.
Mastectomy	Surgical removal of the breast.
Mastication	The act or process of chewing.
Mastitis	Inflammation of the breast.
Mastodynia	Pain in a breast.
Mastoid	Resembling a breast or nipple.
Mastopexy	Surgical fixation of a pendulous or sagging breast.
Mastoplasty	Plastic surgery on the breast.
Mastoscirrhus	Hardening of the mammary gland.
Mastosis	Any disease of the breast.
Maxilla	The upper jawbone.
Megalomania	Delusions of grandeur; unreasonable conviction of one's own greatness.
Melanuria	Black or dark discoloration of the urine.
Metr(a), metr(o)	Combining forms denoting the uterus.
Metritis	Inflammation of the uterus.
Metrocolpocele	Hernial protrusion of the uterus into the vagina.
Metropathy	Any uterine disease.
Metroptosis	Prolapse of the uterus.
Metrorrhagia	Uterine bleeding.
Metrorrhea	A discharge of pus or mucus from the uterus.
Metrostenosis	A narrowing of the uterine cavity.
Mevacor	Brand name for the generic drug lovastatin, used for lowering elevated serum cholesterol.
Micronase	Brand name for glyburide, used to control blood sugar levels in diabetic patients.

Millivolt	1/1000 of a volt.
Molar	A grinding tooth.
Monochromatic	Having only one color.
My(o)	A word element denoting muscle.
Myalgia	Muscle pain.
Myasthenia	Weakness of a muscle.
Mycolog	Brand name for the generic drug nystatin and neomycin sulfate, used for the control of dermatitis.
Myel(o)	A word part denoting the spinal cord or bone marrow.
Myelauxe	Morbid increase in the size of the spinal cord.
Myelocele	Swelling or hernial protrusion of the spinal cord.
Myelocyte	A marrow cell.
Myelogenous	Produced in the bone marrow.
Myelomalacia	Morbid softening of the spinal cord.
Myelophthisis	Wasting of the spinal cord.
Myeloplegia	Paralysis of the spinal cord or spinal paralysis.
Myoblastoma	Tumor of immature muscle cells.
Myocardial	Pertaining to the muscular tissue of the heart.
Myocardiopathy	Disease of the heart muscle.
Myodynia	Muscle pain.
Myokinesis	Movement of muscles.
Myomalacia	Softening of muscles.
Myoplasty	Plastic surgery on a muscle.
Myorrhexis	Rupture or tearing of a muscle.
Myotasis	Stretching of a muscle.
Myx(o)	A combining form denoting mucus or mucous membrane.
Myxadenoma	A tumor with the structure of the mucous glands.
Myxedema	Swelling due to mucus in the tissue.
Myxocystitis	Inflammation of the mucous membrane of the bladder.
Myxoid	Like or resembling a gland.
Myxopoiesis	Making or producing mucus.
Myxorrhea	A flow of mucus.

N

Naphcon A	Eye drop solution used in the treatment of eye irritation or allergic or inflammatory eye problems.
Narcolepsy	An uncontrollable desire for sleep occurring at intervals.
Nas(o)	A combining form denoting the nose.
Nasal	Pertaining to the nose.
Nasograph	An instrument for measuring the nose.
Nasolabial	Pertaining to the nose and lip.

Nasopharyngoscope	An instrument for examination of the nasopharynx.
Nasoscope	A lighted instrument to examine the nose.
Nasoseptal	Pertaining to the nasal septum.
Neoplasm	A new growth.
Neosporin ophthalmic solution	Brand name for polymyxin B-neomycin indicated for the short term treatment of eye infections.
Nephr(o)	A combining form denoting the kidneys.
Nephrapostasis	Abscess of the kidney with supperation.
Nephritis	Inflammation of the kidney.
Nephrohydrosis	An accumulation of water or fluid in the kidney.
Nephrolithiasis	Kidney stones.
Nephrologist (Nephrology)	Specialist in the diagnosis and treatment of kidney disorders.
Nephropathy	Any disease of the kidney.
Nephroptosis	Downward displacement of the kidney.
Neur(o)	A word part denoting the nerves or nervous system.
Neuragmia	The tearing of a nerve.
Neuralgia	Nerve pain.
Neuritis	Inflammation of a nerve.
Neurobiology	The biology of the nervous system.
Neurologist (Neurology)	Deals with disorders of the central nervous system caused by organic disease or injury.
Neuroma	Tumor composed of nerve cells.
Neurooncology	The study of tumors of the nervous system.
Neuropathy	Any disease of the nerves.
Neurosis	An emotional (nervous) disorder characterized by anxiety.
Neurosurgeon (Neurosurgery)	Specializes in the diagnosis and mainly surgical treatment of diseases and disorders of the central nervous system (brain and spinal cord).
Neutrophil	Readily stainable with a neutral stain.
Nitroglycerin	The generic name of a drug used to treat attacks of angina pectoris that are often present in various forms of heart disease. Brand names include Nitro-Dur II, Nitro-bid, and Nitrospan.
Nocturia	Excessive urination at night.
Nolvadex	Brand name for tamoxifen citrate, used for the treatment of female breast cancer.
Nuclear medicine	The branch of medicine concerned with the use of radionuclides in the diagnosis and treatment of disease.

O

Obstetrician (Obstetrics)	Deals with pregnancy, prenatal care and child birth and its aftermath.
Occlusal surface	The chewing or grinding surface of a tooth.

Occlusion	The natural closure and fitting together of the upper and lower jaw.
Octipara	A woman who has had eight pregnancies.
Odontalgia	Toothache.
Oligemia	Deficiency in the volume of blood.
Oligopnea	Retarded or small amount of breathing.
Oniomania	A morbid desire to buy beyond one's realistic needs (shop till you drop).
Onych(o)	A word element denoting the nails.
Onychogenic	Producing nail substance.
Onychoma	Tumor of the nail or nail bed.
Onychomalacia	Softening of the fingernail.
Onychomycosis	Fungus condition of the nails.
Onychophagia	Habitual biting of the nails.
Onychoptosis	Falling off of the nail.
Onychorrhexis	Splitting or rupture of the nail.
Onychosis	A disease of the nail.
Oophor(o)	A word part denoting the ovaries.
Oophorectomy	Excision or removal of an ovary.
Oophoritis	Inflammation of an ovary.
Oophorocystosis	The formation of an ovarian cyst.
Oophoroma	Tumor of the ovary.
Oophoroplasty	Plastic surgery on an ovary.
Oophorrhagia	Hemorrhage or bleeding of an ovary.
Oophorostomy	The making of an opening into an ovarian cyst to provide drainage.
Ophthalm(o)	A combining form denoting the eye.
Ophthalmocopia	Eyestrain or weariness of the eyes.
Ophthalmodonesis	A trembling motion of the eye.
Ophthalmologist (Ophthalmology)	A physician who deals with all areas involving the eye.
Ophthalmology	Study or science of what is known of the eye.
Ophthalmomalacia	Abnormal softness of the eye or eyeball.
Ophthalmometer	An instrument for measuring the eye.
Ophthalmomyitis	Inflammation of the muscles that move the eyeball.
Ophthalmoplegia	Paralysis of the eye muscle.
Ophthalmoscope	An instrument to examine the eye.
Ophthalmosteresis	Loss of an eye.
Oral pathology	The branch of dentistry concerned with diseases of the teeth and mouth.
Oral surgery	The branch of dentistry that involves operative procedures of the teeth and mouth.
Organidin	Brand name for iodinated glycerol, prescribed as an expectorant in respiratory conditions such as bronchitis.

Orthodontics	The branch of dentistry that deals with the prevention and correction of irregularities of teeth and malocclusion.
Orthopedic surgeon, (Orthopedic surgery) orthopedist	Deals with the diagnosis and mainly surgical treatment of the musculoskeletal system.
Orthopnea	Inability to breathe unless one is in an upright position.
Oste(o)	A word element denoting the bones.
Osteitis	Inflammation of the bone.
Osteoclasis	Surgical fracture of refracture of a bone.
Osteofibroma	Tumor composed of fibrous and osseous material.
Osteogenesis	Producing bone.
Osteohypertrophy	A condition characterized by overgrowth of bone.
Osteolysis	Softening, destruction and absorption of bony tissue.
Osteomalacia	Softening of the bone.
Osteoporosis	Reduction in the quantity of bone or atrophy of skeletal tissue.
Ot(o)	A combining form denoting the ear.
Otalgia	Earache or pain in the ear.
Otitis	Inflammation of the ear.
Otoblennorrhea	Mucus discharge from the ear.
Otolaryngologist (Otolaryngology)	Specialist in the diagnosis and treatment of disorders of the ear, nose and throat.
Otologist	Specialist in treating ear disorders.
Otomycosis	Fungus infection of the ear.
Otopyosis	Formation of pus in the ear.
Otorrhea	A discharge from the ear.
Otosclerosis	A new formation of spongy bone in the ear.
Ovari(o)	A combining form denoting the ovaries.
Ovariocele	Hernial protrusion or tumor of an ovary.
Ovariocentesis	Surgical puncture of an ovary.
Ovariocyesis	Ovarian pregnancy.
Ovariodysneuria	Neural pain in an ovary.
Ovariopathy	Ovarian disease.
Ovariorrhexis	Rupture of an ovary.
Ovariosalpingectomy	Removal of the ovary and oviduct.
Ovariotubal	Pertaining to the ovary and uterine tubes.

P

Pachyblepharon	Thickening of the eyelid.
Palate	The roof of the mouth.
Pancreat(o)	A combining form denoting relationship to the pancreas.
Pancreatectomy	Surgical removal of the pancreas.
Pancreathelcosis	Ulceration of the pancreas.

Pancreatic Pertaining to the pancreas.

Pancreatitis Inflammation of the pancreas.

Pancreatoid Like or resembling the pancreas.

Pancreatolith Stone or calculus in the pancreas.

Pancreatopathy A disease of the pancreas.

Pancreatolysis Destruction of pancreatic tissue.

Panhysterectomy Total removal of the uterus and cervix (total hysterectomy).

Pathologist (Pathology) Deals primarily with the diagnosis of disease.

Pediatrician (Pediatrics) Specializes in the diagnosis of diseases of children.

Pedodontics The branch of dentistry that treats dental conditions in children.

Pedophilia A morbid sexual perversion toward children.

Penicillin Ampicillin. The generic name for a variety of brand names such as V-Cillin K, Ledercillin VK and Pen Vee K, used to treat a variety of infections.

Pentachromic Pertaining to or exhibiting five colors.

Pericarditis Inflammation of the membrane around the heart.

Pericardium The fibroserous sac surrounding the heart.

Permanent teeth The teeth of adults.

Persantine Brand name for dipyridamole, indicated to increase the blood flow following surgical cardiac valve replacement.

Pharmacologist One who specializes in the study of the action of drugs.

Pharyng(o) A word part denoting the pharynx.

Pharyngemphraxis Obstruction of the pharynx.

Pharyngitis Inflammation of the pharynx.

Pharyngonasal Pertaining to the nose and pharynx.

Pharyngosalpingitis Inflammation of the pharynx and eustachian tube.

Pharyngoscope Instrument used to examine the pharynx.

Pharyngostenosis Narrowing of the pharynx.

Pharyngoxerosis Dryness of the pharynx.

Phenergan Brand name for promethazine hydrochloride alcohol, a syrup prescribed for the relief of nasal and chest congestion.

Phenobarbital The generic name for various brand name drugs prescribed as a sleep-producing agent and sedative.

Phil(ia) Word ending denoting love or attraction to.

Phleb(o) A word part denoting the vein or veins.

Phlebitis Inflammation of a vein.

Phlebodynamics Laws and principles governing blood pressure.

Phleboplasty Plastic surgery on a vein.

Phleborrhagia Excessive bleeding from a vein.

Phleborrhaphy Suture or surgical repair of a vein.

Phlebosclerosis Hardening of the walls of the veins.

Phlebostenosis	Narrowing or constriction of a vein.
Phlebotomy	Incision into a vein.
Photoretinitis	Inflammation of the retina due to exposure to intense light.
Physiatrist (Physical medicine and rehabilitation)	Specializes in the treatment of disease by the use of physical agents such as heat, light, water and mechanical apparatus.
Plaquenil	Brand name for the generic drug hydroxychloroquine sulfate, prescribed for the treatment of acute or chronic rheumatoid arthritis and other disorders.
Plastic surgeon (Plastic surgery)	Deals with the restoration or repairs of defects of the human body.
Pleocytosis	Presence of a greater number of cells than normal.
Pleur(o)	A combining form indicating the pleura (the membrane lining the chest cavity and covering the lungs).
Pleural	Of or relating to the pleura.
Pleuralgia	Pain in the pleural region.
Pleurocele	Herniation of the lung tissue of the pleura.
Pleurocentesis	Surgical puncture or tap of the pleura.
Pleuroclysis	The flushing out of the pleural cavity.
Pleurorrhea	Effusion of fluid into the pleura.
Pleurotomy	Incision into the pleura.
Pnea	A word ending denoting breathing, air or gas.
Pneum(a), pneum(o), pneum(ato), pneumon(o)	A combining form denoting lungs, respiration, air or gas.
Pneumocentesis	Surgical puncture for aspiration of the lung.
Pneumoconiosis	A disease caused by dust or other particulates in the lungs.
Pneumodynamics	The dynamics of the respiratory system.
Pneumoencephalography	Radiographic films of the brain utilizing injections of air or gas.
Pneumomelanosis	A blackening of the lungs as from coal dust.
Pneumonitis	Inflammation of the lung.
Pneumonography	X-ray of the lung.
Pneumothorax	Accumulation of air in the chest cavity.
Poliomyelitis	Inflammation of the gray matter of the spinal cord.
Polychromatophilia	The quality of being stainable with various stains or colors.
Polycythemia	Increase in the number of red cells in the blood.
Polydipsia	Excessive thirst.
Polyphagia	Excessive or overeating (bulimia).
Polyuria	Excessive secretion of urine.
Pontic	The portion of a dental bridge that replaces a tooth.
Postmortem	Occurring or performed after death.
Prednisone	The generic name of a drug prescribed as an antiinflammatory agent.

Premarin	Brand name for conjugated estrogens, generally prescribed as estrogen replacement therapy.
Preventive medicine	That branch of study of medicine that aims at the prevention of disease.
Proct(o)	A word element denoting the rectum or anus.
Proctatresia	Anal atresia, absence of a proper rectal opening.
Proctocele	Hernial protrusion of the rectum.
Proctologist (Proctology)	Specializes in the diagnosis and treatment of disorders of the rectum and sigmoid colon.
Proctopexy	Surgical fixation or fastening of the rectum.
Proctoptosis	Prolapse or falling of the rectum.
Proctorrhea	A mucoserous discharge from the rectum.
Proctoscopy	Examination of the rectum by the use of a proctoscope.
Propine	Brand name for dipivefrin hydrochloride, used to control internal eye pressure in glaucoma.
Propranolol	The generic name for inderal, a potent drug which is prescribed for various heart conditions such as angina pectoris.
Prosthesis	The replacement of part of the body by an artificial part such as dentures.
Prosthodontics	Dentistry that deals with the replacement of natural teeth with prosthetics.
Protoplasia	The primary formation of tissue.
Proventil	Brand name for the generic drug albuterol, prescribed for the relief of breathing difficulty.
Pseudocyesis	False pregnancy.
Psych(o)	A word part denoting the mind or mental faculties.
Psychasthenia	A term to denote a functional personality disorder literally translated as mental weakness.
Psychataxia	Mental confusion, inability to fix the attention.
Psychiatrist (Psychiatry)	Deals with functional disorders of the mind.
Psychogenic	Originating or developing in the mind.
Psychology	The branch of medicine that studies the mind.
Psychoneurosis	A mental or behavioral disorder which presents symptoms of functional nervous disease.
Psychophylaxis	Preventing mental illness.
Psychosomatic	Pertaining to the mind-body relationship.
Psychotherapy	Treatment of emotional, behavioral and emotional disorders.
Pulmonary disease	The branch of medicine that treats diseases of the chest and thorax.
Pulp	The soft tissue that fills the inside of teeth.
Purpuriferous	Producing a purple pigment.
Pyel(o)	A word part denoting the pelvis of the kidney.
Pyelectasis	Dilatation of the kidney pelvis.

Pyelitis	Inflammation of the pelvis of the kidney.
Pyelocystitis	Inflammation of the renal pelvis and bladder.
Pyelography	Roentgenographic study of the kidney and renal collecting system.
Pyelolithotomy	The operation of removing a renal calculus from the pelvis of the kidney.
Pyelonephritis	Inflammation of the kidney and its pelvis.
Pyelophlebitis	Inflammation of the veins of the renal pelvis.
Pyeloscopy	Examination or observation of kidney pelvis via a fluoroscope.
Pyridium	Brand name for the generic drug phenazopyridine hydrochloride, prescribed for the relief of urinary pain, urgency, frequency, etc.
Pyromania	A morbid compulsion to set fires.
Pyuria	Presence of pus in the urine.

Q

Quadruped	Four footed, such as many animals.
Quinamm	Brand name for quinine sulfate, prescribed for nocturnal leg muscle cramps.
Quinidine	The generic name for Quinaglute, used to increase contractability of the heart muscle. Also used to treat irregular rhythm of the heart.
Quinquecuspid	A tooth having five points or cusps.

R

Rachiocentesis	Spinal (lumbar) puncture.
Radiologist (Radiology)	Specializes in the diagnostic and therapeutic use of radiant energy.
Reglan	Brand name for metoclopramide hydrochloride, prescribed for the relief of gastro-intestinal symptoms in some diabetic patients.
Retin-A	Brand name for the generic drug tretinoin, used in the treatment of some kinds of acne.
Retractor	An instrument to draw back and hold the edges of a wound.
Retroflexed	Bent backwards.
Rheumatologist (Rheumatology)	Specializes in the diagnosis and treatment of rheumatism.
Rhin(o)	A combining form denoting the nose.
Rhinesthesia	Pertaining to the sense of smell.
Rhinitis	Inflammation of the nose.
Rhinocheiloplasty	Plastic surgery on the lip and nose.
Rhinodynia	Pain in the nose or nasal area.
Rhinolith	A stone or concretion of the nose.
Rhinomycosis	Fungus infection of the nose.
Rhinorrhagia	Nosebleed.
Root	The portion of a tooth that is within the socket.

Root canal	The space within the root of the tooth containing the pulp.
Rubeosis	Redness of an area.

S

Salping(o)	A word part denoting the uterine (fallopian) tubes or auditory (eustachian) tubes.
Salpingemphraxis	Obstruction of the uterine or eustachian tube.
Salpingitis	Inflammation of the uterine tube or canal.
Salpingocele	The formation of an ovarian cyst.
Salpingocyesis	Tubal pregnancy.
Salpingography	Visual examination of the uterine tube.
Salpingo-oophorectomy	Excision of the ovary and uterine tube.
Salpingorrhagia	Hemorrhage from a fallopian tube.
Salpingorrhaphy	Suture or surgical repair of the uterine tube.
Salpingoscopy	Visual examination of the uterine tube.
Salpingotomy	Surgical incision into the uterine tube.
Saprophyte	An organism, such as bacteria, living upon decaying matter.
Sarc(o)	A word element denoting flesh or connective tissue.
Sarcoblast	Primitive or immature cell which develops into connective tissue.
Sarcoid	Like or resembling flesh.
Sarcolysis	Destruction or dissolution of flesh.
Sarcoma	Tumor of fleshy or connective tissue.
Sarcomphalocele	A fleshy tumor of the umbilicus.
Sarcopoietic	Producing flesh or muscle.
Sarcosepsis	Sepsis due to presence of bacteria in the tissue.
Sarcostosis	Ossification of fleshy tissue.
Semicoma	A stupor from which the patient may be aroused.
Septra	Brand name of the generic drug trimethoprim sulfamethoxazole, used in the treatment of types of urinary infections.
Sinemet	Brand name for levodopa, which is prescribed for the treatment of patients with Parkinson's disease.
Sperm(a), sperm(ato), sperm(i), sperm(o)	A word element denoting a seed, usually the male generative element (semen).
Spermatism	Promoting the secretion of semen.
Spermatocyte	A sperm cell.
Spermatopoietic	Pertaining to a condition in which semen is produced or developed.
Spermatorrhea	An involuntary discharge of semen without organism.
Spermatoschesis	Suppression of the discharge of semen.
Spermicide	An agent that is destructive to spermatozoa.
Spermophlebectasia	Dilatation or varicosity of the spermatic veins.
Sphygm(o)	A word part denoting the pulse or blood pressure.
Sphygmogram	Record or tracing of the pulse.

Sphygmoid	Like or resembling the pulse.
Sphygmology	The study of science of what is known of the pulse.
Sphygmomanometer	An instrument for measuring the blood pressure.
Sphygmopalpation	Palpating or feeling the pulse.
Sphygmoscopy	Examination of the pulse.
Splen(o)	A combing form denoting the spleen.
Splenatrophy	Atrophy or wasting of the spleen.
Splenectomy	Excision or removal of the spleen.
Splenocele	Herniation or swelling of the spleen.
Splenohepatomegaly	Enlargement of the spleen and liver.
Splenoncus	Tumor of the spleen.
Splenophrenic	Pertaining to the spleen and diaphragm.
Splenorrhagia	Bleeding or hemorrhage of the spleen.
Spondyl(o)	A word element denoting the vertebra or spinal column.
Spondylalgia	Pain in a vertebra.
Spondylexarthrosis	A condition in which a vertebra is out of its joint or is dislocated.
Spondylitis	Inflammation of a vertebra.
Spondylolisthesis	Slipping of one vertebra over another.
Spondylomalacia	Softening of a vertebra.
Spondylopyosis	Suppuration of one or more of the vertebral bodies.
Spondylotherapy	Treatment applied to the spinal region.
Sublingual	Situated beneath the tongue.
Supernumerary tooth	A tooth in excess of the regular number.
Supratympanic	Situated above the tympanum.
Surgeon (Surgery)	Specializes in treating pathologic or traumatic conditions by operative procedures.
Syndesm(o)	A word element denoting ligaments.
Syndesmectopia	Displacement of a ligament.
Syndesmitis	Inflammation of a ligament.
Syndesmoma	A connective tissue (ligament) tumor.
Syndesmopexy	Operative fixation of a dislocation using the joint ligaments.
Syndesmoplasty	Plastic surgery on a ligament.
Syndesmorrhaphy	Suture or repair of a ligament.
Syndesmotomy	The cutting of a ligament.
Synthroid	Brand name for levothyroxine sodium, prescribed for patients who have a decreased amount of thyroid hormone production.

T

Tachycardia	Excessive rapidity of the action of the heart, usually in the pulse rate.
Tachypnea	Abnormally fast rate of breathing.

Tagamet	Brand name for the generic drug cimetidine, prescribed to lower acid secretion in the stomach; indicated in the treatment of duodenal ulcers.
Tegretol	Brand name for carbamazepine, used to control epilepsy and also the pain from trigeminal neuralgia.
Temporomandibular joint	The joint, just ahead of the ear, which swings the lower jaw open.
Ten(o), tend(o)	A word part denoting a tendon.
Tendoplasty	Plastic surgery on a tendon.
Tenodesis	Tendon fixation.
Tenodynia	Pain in a tendon.
Tenonectomy	Excision of a part of a tendon.
Tenorrhaphy	The union of a divided tendon by suture.
Tenosynovitis	Inflammation of a tendon together with its sheath.
Tenotomy	The cutting of a tendon as for strabismus or clubfoot.
Tertian	Recurring every third day.
Tetradactyly	The condition of having four digits on the hands or feet.
Theo-Dur	Brand name for theophylline, which is used in the treatment of patients suffering from respiratory diseases such as asthma, bronchitis and emphysema.
Thorac(o)	A word element denoting the chest or thorax.
Throracentesis	Surgical puncture of the chest.
Thoracic surgeon (Thoracic surgery)	Specializes in the diagnosis and treatment (mainly surgical) of disorders of the organs of the thoracic cavity, generally the heart and lungs.
Thoracocyllosis	A deformity of the chest.
Thoracodynia	Pain in the chest region.
Thoracomyodynia	Pain in the muscles of the chest.
Thoracoplasty	Plastic surgery of the chest.
Thoracoscopy	Examination of the chest.
Thoracotomy	Incision into the chest.
Thromb(o)	A combining form indicating a blood clot or thrombus.
Thrombectomy	Removal or excision of a thrombus.
Thromboarteritis	Inflammation of an artery with a clot present.
Thromboclasis	The breaking up or dissolution of a thrombus.
Thrombocyte	A clotting cell.
Thrombocytopenia	Decrease in the number of clotting cells.
Thrombocytosis	An unusually large number of thrombocytes (platelets) in the blood.
Thrombogenic	Producing a clot or thrombus.
Thromboid	Like or resembling a clot.
Thrombopathy	Disease involving clotting cells.
Thrombophlebitis	Inflammation of a vein in which a clot is present.
Thrombopoiesis	The formation of clots or thrombi.

Thrombosis	A condition in which a clot is present.
Thyr(o)	A combining form denoting the thyroid gland.
Thyrocele	A tumor of the thyroid gland; a goiter.
Thyrogenous	Originating in the thyroid gland.
Thyroiditis	Inflammation of the thyroid gland.
Thyropenia	Decreased or deficient activity of the thyroid gland.
Thyroptosis	Downward displacement of the thyroid gland.
Thyrotoxicosis	A disease (toxic) resulting from overactivity of the thyroid gland.
Tigan	Brand name for trimethobenzamide hydrochloride, prescribed the control nausea and vomiting.
Timoptic	Brand name for timolol maleate, prescribed for the treatment of glaucoma. It lowers elevated eye pressure.
Trache(o)	A word part denoting the trachea or windpipe.
Tracheitis	Inflammation of the trachea.
Trachelodynia	Pain in the neck.
Tracheopathy	Any disease of the trachea.
Tracheoplasty	Plastic surgery on the trachea.
Tracheopyosis	Suppurative inflammation of the trachea.
Tracheorrhaphy	Surgical repair or suture of the trachea.
Tracheostenosis	Narrowing of the trachea.
Tracheotomy	Incision into the trachea.
Trental	Brand name for pentoxifylline, used to increase blood flow in patients with muscle pain.
Trich(o)	A word part indicating the hair or the capillary (hair-like) vessels.
Trichalgia	Pain when the hair is touched.
Trichoclasis	Abnormal brittleness of the hair.
Trichogenous	Promoting growth of hair.
Trichoglossia	A hairy condition of the tongue.
Trichomycosis	Fungus infection of the hair.
Trichopathy	A disease of the hair.
Trichoschisis	Splitting of the hair.
Triorchidism	The condition of having three testes.

U

Ultrasonic	Having a frequency above sound.
Unilateral	Pertaining to or affecting only one side.
Urecholine	Brand name for bethanechol chloride, used for the treatment of postoperative and postpartum nonobstructive urinary retention.
Uria	A word ending (suffix) having to do with urine or urination.
Urologist (Urology)	Specializes in the diagnosis and treatment of disorders and diseases of the urinary system in both sexes and the male genital system.

V

Valium	Brand name for diazepam, used for the relief of anxiety and tension.
Vasectomy	Surgical removal of the ductus deferens or a portion of it.
Vas(o)	A word part denoting a vessel or duct.
Vasography	X-ray picture or roentgenogram of blood vessels.
Vasomotor	Affecting the movement and size of a vessel.
Vasorrhaphy	Suture of a vessel or the ductus deferens.
Vasosection	The cutting of a vessel.
Vasospasm	Contraction of a vessel.
Vasotec	Brand name for the drug enalapril maleate, used in the treatment of high blood pressure.
Voltaren	Brand name for the generic drug diclofenac sodium, prescribed for the relief of acute and chronic symptoms of arthritis.

X

Xanthochromic	Denoting a yellow discoloration of the spinal fluid.

Z

Zantac	Brand name for the generic drug ranitidine hydrochloride, used in the treatment of patients with duodenal and gastric ulcers.
Zoophobia	Abnormal fear or dread of animals.
Zovirax	Brand name for the generic drug acyclovir, used in the treatment of genital herpes.
Zygomatic arch	The "cheekbone."

Index

A

B

C

D

E

F

G

M

N

O

P

Q

R

S

T

U

V

W

X

Z